Platinum Vignettes™

Ultra-high-yield Clinical Case Scenarios for USMLE Step 1

Anatomy & Embryology

PLATINUM VIGNETTES™
ULTRA-HIGH-YIELD CLINICAL CASE SCENARIOS FOR USMLE STEP 1

Anatomy & Embryology

ADAM BROCHERT, MD
Resident
Department of Radiology
Medical College of Georgia
Memorial Health University Medical Center
Savannah, Georgia

Hanley & Belfus
An imprint of Elsevier

HANLEY & BELFUS
An Imprint of Elsevier

The Curtis Center
Independence Square West
Philadelphia, Pennsylvania 19106

Note to the reader: Although the information in this book has been carefully reviewed for correctness of dosage and indications, neither the author nor the publisher can accept any legal responsibility for any errors or omissions that may be made. Neither the publisher nor the author makes any warranty, expressed or implied, with respect to the material contained herein. Before prescribing any drug, the reader must review the manufacturer's current product information (package inserts) for accepted indications, absolute dosage recommendations, and other information pertinent to the safe and effective use of the product described. This is especially important when drugs are given in combination or as an adjunct to other forms of therapy.

Library of Congress Control Number: 2003101727

PLATINUM VIGNETTES™: ANATOMY & EMBRYOLOGY ISBN 1-56053-581-4

Printed in the United States

Last digit is the print number: 9 8 7 6 5 4 3 2 1

INTRODUCTION

Case scenarios are a great way to review for the USMLE Step 1 exam. The current exam format has a high percentage of questions that center on a case format or patient presentation. Practicing this format and being familiar with the majority of the classic "guaranteed to be on the exam" case scenarios gives the examinee an obvious, clear-cut advantage. The *Platinum Vignettes*™ series was written to give you that advantage.

For the Step 1 exam, you need to be familiar with both normal human biology and pathophysiology, but examinees are increasingly being asked questions about diagnostic tests and treatments, topics previously reserved for the Step 2 exam. After sifting through the history, physical exam findings, and various tests in a case presentation, you are expected to know the diagnosis and, furthermore, understand the mechanism of the underlying pathophysiology and why common treatments are effective.

The format of this series is to present a case scenario or clinical vignette on one side of the page, with the explanation of the diagnosis or issue, pathophysiology, diagnostic tests, and treatments on the other side of the page. This allows the reader to "guess" before reading about the patient's condition. The reader is advised not only to guess the diagnosis, but also to postulate on the mechanisms of the disease and any treatments, which confirmatory test to order, what therapy to give, and what to "watch out" for.

Important words or phrases ("buzzwords") are set in bold type. This is the material most commonly asked about on the exam, and/or this information is important to help you distinguish one condition from another. Because the *Platinum Vignettes*™ format is designed for review of material that was "supposed to be" learned during the first 2 years of medical school, further reading is advised if a topic or buzzword is unfamiliar. Remember, buzzwords are rarely helpful unless you know what they mean!

Every attempt was made to give the most current, up-to-date information on every topic tackled in this volume and every volume in the series, but medicine is a rapidly changing field. Remember, though, that most board questions are at least a few years old by the time you see them on your Step 1 exam.

Good luck!

Adam Brochert, MD

NOTE: *A standard table of contents, with cases listed by diagnosis, would give you too much of a head start on solving each patient scenario. Challenge yourself! When ready, you can turn to the detailed Case Index at the back of this book (page 109).*

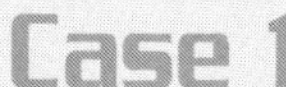

Case 1

Anatomy & Embryology

History

A 42-year-old woman presents with headache and confusion. Her past medical history is unremarkable, and the patient takes no medications.

Physical Exam

Vital signs are normal. No focal neurologic deficits are appreciated, but the patient is confused and disoriented.

Tests

MRI of the brain (see figure): sagittal (*top*) and axial (*bottom*).

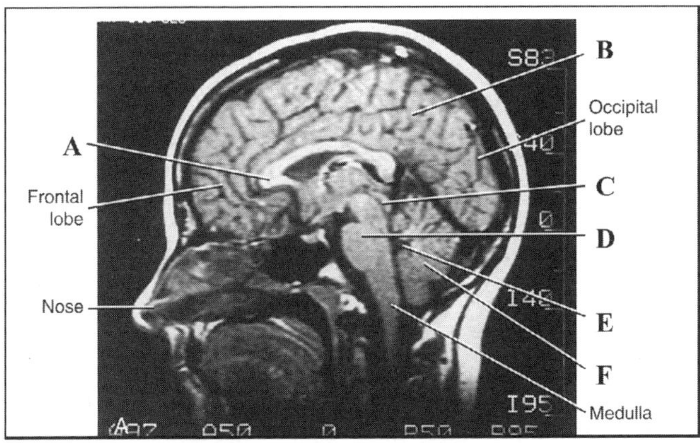

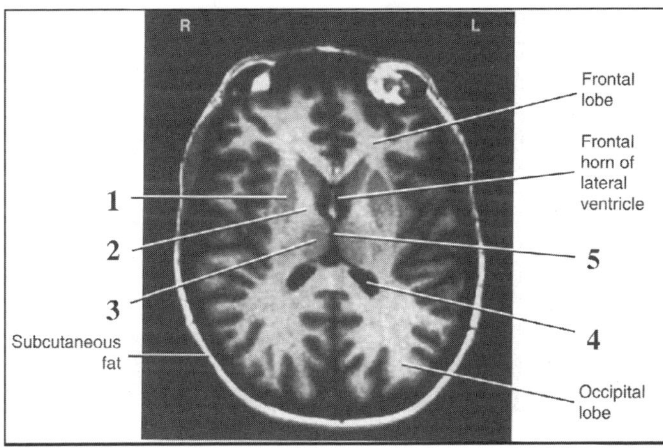

Questions

- What are the major structures labeled *A* through *F* in the sagittal, midline MRI image?
- What are the structures labeled *1* through *5* in the axial MRI image?

Discussion

MRI has become the most sensitive and specific imaging modality for most conditions of the central nervous system and can provide images along any axis—axial, sagittal, and coronal images routinely are acquired. MRI images are also useful for testing a medical student's understanding of neuroanatomy.

Anatomy

In the sagittal image, the parietal lobe (labeled *B* in the figure) is shown between the frontal and occipital lobes. Communication between hemispheres is facilitated by the **corpus callosum** (*A*). Below the cerebral hemispheres lies the top of the brainstem, which contains the *thalamus* (labeled *3* in the axial image) and *hypothalamus*. Caudal to these are the *midbrain* (at the level of *C*), *pons* (*D*) and *medulla*. The cerebellum (*F*) is posterior to the brainstem and lies beneath the **tentorium cerebelli.**

The ventricular system includes the paired off-midline *lateral ventricles* (the *atrium* of the left lateral ventricle is labeled *4*), which lie within the cerebral hemispheres. The lateral ventricles connect with the midline *third ventricle* (*5*), which separates the thalami, by way of the **foramina of Monro.** The **aqueduct of Sylvius** (*C*) connects the third ventricle to the *fourth ventricle* (*E*) and lies between the cerebral peduncle (specifically the *tegmentum*) and *tectum* (primarily contains the superior and inferior colliculi) of the midbrain.

Many of the fibers heading to and from the cerebral hemispheres travel through the compact **internal capsule** (*2*), which runs between the *caudate* nucleus (adjacent to frontal horn of lateral ventricle) and the more medial *putamen* (*1*) and *globus pallidus;* the latter two sometimes are grouped and called the **lentiform nucleus.**

More High-Yield Facts

Cerebrospinal fluid (CSF) is secreted primarily by the choroid plexus, which is located in each of the ventricles. CSF can exit the fourth ventricle, which lies between the pons and cerebellum, via the *m*idline foramen of ***M*agendie** or the *l*ateral foramen of ***L*uschka.** After leaving the fourth ventricle, CSF flows in the *subarachnoid space,* bathing the spinal cord and brain. The **arachnoid villi** are protrusions of pia-arachnoid through the dura mater and into the dural venous sinuses that allow CSF diffusion into the bloodstream. This is good because CSF is produced at a daily rate of 500 mL, when there is normally space for only 150 mL.

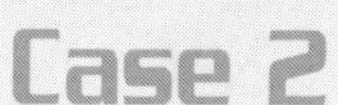

Case 2

Anatomy & Embryology

History

An 8-month-old African-American girl is brought into your office for irritability and low-grade fever. The patient's caretaker reports that, as far as she knows, the infant has been healthy and takes no medications. The caretaker is watching the infant for her cousin.

History

The infant was born without difficulty. There is a history of anemia in the mother and father's family, although neither of the patient's parents has anemia. The patient has no recent history of travel, toxic exposure, or illness.

Physical Exam

The patient is healthy-appearing but irritable, with normal height and weight. You note mild pallor of the mucous membranes and painful and swollen hands and feet (dactylitis).

Tests

Hemoglobin: low
Hematocrit: low
Platelets: normal
Prothrombin time: normal
Peripheral blood smear: see figure

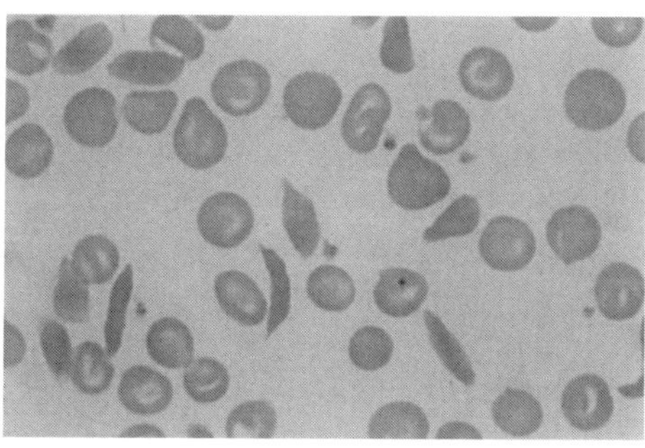

Questions

- What does the peripheral blood smear in the figure reveal?
- What causes this condition?

Topic

Sickle cell anemia, also known as sickle cell disease (SCD)

Discussion

The peripheral blood smear reveals classic-appearing sickled red blood cells (RBCs). SCD is the classic hereditary hemoglobinopathy. These disorders (e.g., thalassemia) result in the production of structurally abnormal hemoglobin. In SCD, which is autosomal recessive, a mutation in the β-globin chain (classically a point mutation that causes a substitution of valine for glutamic acid in the sixth position of β-hemoglobin) results in the formation of hemoglobin S.

Hemoglobin S undergoes a conformational change when it becomes deoxygenated, causing aggregation of hemoglobin S proteins and the classic sickled appearance of RBCs. The end result is a hemolytic anemia, as sickled cells are sequestered in the sinusoids of the spleen and destroyed. Average RBC survival decreases from 120 days to 20 days.

Findings

When illness, dehydration, or a fall in pH occur, RBCs in patients with SCD may become sickled. RBC destruction in the spleen causes **chronic anemia** (with an appropriately *increased* ***reticulocyte*** *count,* assuming the bone marrow functions properly), hyperbilirubinemia, and (pigment) **gallstones.** Patients also can have painful "crises" resulting from vascular occlusion or infarct vital tissues (e.g., bone or kidney infarct, **stroke,** "chest syndrome," *priapism,* **dactylitis** [painful finger or toe swelling] or intestinal ischemia). The peripheral smear is classic, revealing sickled RBCs.

Treatment

Patients often do not have symptoms until 4 to 6 months of life, when fetal hemoglobin declines and the amount of hemoglobin S increases. Currently, treatment is largely supportive, and hydration can help reverse RBC sickling in some cases. Because the condition is autosomal recessive, the parents in this case probably have a 25% chance of having another affected offspring because neither has SCD (both likely "silent" carriers—said to have **sickle cell trait**).

More High-Yield Facts

Patients initially have splenomegaly but eventually "autoinfarct" their spleen and have splenic dysfunction, increasing the risk of infection with **encapsulated** bacteria (e.g., *Haemophilus influenzae, Streptococcus pneumoniae, Neisseria meningitidis*).

A classic cause of **osteomyelitis** in SCD patients is *Salmonella.*

An aplastic crisis (acute bone marrow failure) in SCD patients can be caused by **parvovirus B19** infection.

Anatomy & Embryology

History

A 20-year-old woman comes to your office worried that she is abnormal because she has never menstruated. The patient has a history of coarctation of the aorta, which was repaired when she was 6 months old because of its severity. Otherwise the patient has no significant past medical history. She takes no regular medications. Family history is unremarkable. The patient has never been sexually active.

Physical Exam

The patient is < 5 feet tall and has some webbing of her neck. You also note a low posterior hairline and broad chest with widely spaced nipples. No abnormal heart sounds are appreciated, and the lungs are clear to auscultation. She has prepubescent development of secondary sex characteristics. On pelvic exam, the uterus is small. No neurologic deficits are appreciated.

Tests

Hemoglobin: normal
Liver function tests: normal
Follicle-stimulating hormone (FSH): elevated
Thyroid-stimulating hormone: normal
Pelvic ultrasound: small "streak" ovaries noted bilaterally
Buccal smear: no Barr bodies identified

Questions

- What condition does this patient have?
- What is a Barr body?

Topic Turner syndrome (TS)

Discussion

TS is a chromosomal disorder affecting **females.** It is classically due to a missing X chromosome (*45, XO* karyotype), although mosaicism and isochromosomes, deletions, and ring forms of one X chromosome also can cause TS. The lack of critical X chromosome genes results in a **lack of adult sexual development.** Associated developmental abnormalities are frequent and classic on boards: **aortic coarctation, short stature** (< 5 feet tall), *low posterior hairline, webbing of the neck, broad chest with widely spaced nipples,* and *cubitus valgus* (a wide carrying angle at the elbow).

The most common causes for *aneuploidy* (wrong number of chromosomes) are **nondisjunction,** which is when a chromosomal or chromatid pair fails to separate during the first or second meiotic division, and **anaphase lag.** In the latter, one chromosome (meiosis) or chromatid (mitosis) moves too slow for the group and is excluded from the nucleus of a cell.

Findings

Classic TS patient presentations are for primary **amenorrhea** (patients who have not menstruated by age 16) or **infertility,** although many are diagnosed prenatally or shortly after birth. Classic physical exam findings include perinatal swelling in the neck from a **cystic hygroma** (benign cystic growth, classically in the neck) and lack of adult sexual development, including sparse pubic hair, lack of breast development, small uterus, and *"streak" ovaries* (i.e., small, nonfunctional ovaries). Elevated *gonadotropin* (e.g., FSH) levels occur and stem from attempts by the hypothalamus and pituitary gland to stimulate the ovaries (a form of premature menopause).

Treatment

Treatment may be needed for embryologic defects (e.g., coarctation, cystic hygroma). Intelligence is usually normal, but the risk of mental retardation is increased.

More High-Yield Facts

A Barr body is a condensed mass of chromatin representing an inactivated X-chromosome. Males (XY) and TS patients (XO) have no Barr bodies, but normal women (XX) have Barr bodies, as only those with more than one X chromosome (including males with Klinefelter syndrome [XXY]) can "afford" to have one X chromosome inactivated. Only roughly half of cells have Barr bodies in those with more than one X chromosome.

Case 4

Anatomy & Embryology

History

A mother brings in her newborn because the infant is "blue." The infant was born 1 week ago at home without difficulty. This is the infant's first physician visit. The mother states that the infant has a dusky blue hue on his skin, especially around the face and lips. She wants to know if this is normal or not. There is no significant family history.

Physical Exam

The infant is cyanotic, most notably in the facial area and mucous membranes. You hear a loud heart murmur along the left sternal border during systole. On testing, the infant is hypoxic.

Tests

Hemoglobin: normal

MRI of the heart (see figure): right ventricular hypertrophy and an abnormal appearance of the cardiovascular structures

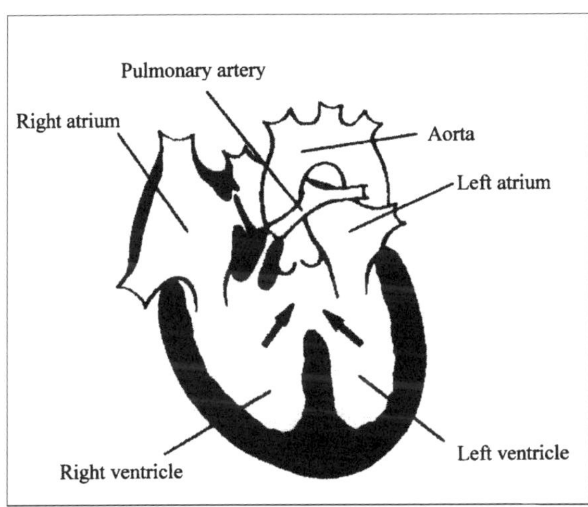

Questions

- What is the name of this congenital heart defect?
- Describe the components of this anomaly.
- Why is the child cyanotic?
- Can you name any other congenital cardiac defects that cause cyanosis?

Topic Tetralogy of Fallot (TOF)

Discussion

The cause of TOF is not well understood, but it is composed of four (*tetra* = 4) classic abnormalities: **pulmonic stenosis, ventricular septal defect** (VSD), **right ventricular hypertrophy,** and an **"overriding" aorta** (aorta straddles the VSD and receives blood from both ventricles).

Because of stenosis and underdevelopment of the pulmonary outflow tract, blood has trouble traveling from the right ventricle to the lungs (contributing to the right ventricular hypertrophy as the heart tries to overcome the increased resistance). The VSD (*arrows* in the figure point to the absent superior portion of the interventricular septum) and overriding aorta lead to mixing of deoxygenated and oxygenated blood from the right and left ventricles. The resulting cyanosis, which is usually present, can range from mild to severe.

Findings

Children are classically **cyanotic** (TOF is the most common cause of cyanotic congenital heart disease after the age of 1 or 2 years) and **hypoxic.** They also have a **systolic heart murmur** from their VSD, a pansystolic murmur best heard along the lower left sternal border.

Diagnosis & Treatment

The diagnosis is made with imaging, usually a cardiac ultrasound (echocardiogram). Treatment is surgical correction.

More High-Yield Facts

The causes of cyanotic congenital heart disease (the **5 Ts**):
1. ***T**ransposition of the great arteries* (most common cause at birth): The aorta arises from the right ventricle and the pulmonary artery arises from the left ventricle. A VSD, patent foramen ovale, or patent ductus arteriosus (shunt) generally must coexist to allow mixture of oxygenated and unoxygenated blood.
2. ***T**ricuspid atresia:* Tricuspid valve orifice fails to develop and is occluded. A shunt generally must be present, as in transposition.
3. ***T**runcus arteriosus:* Defect in the aorticopulmonary septum, which normally divides the embryologic truncus into the aorta and pulmonary artery, results in a single artery receiving blood from both ventricles; this usually is accompanied by a defect in the upper ventricular septum.
4. ***T**otal anomalous pulmonary venous return:* No pulmonary veins drain into the left atrium; rather the veins drain into the systemic circulation (e.g., inferior vena cava).
5. ***T**etralogy of Fallot

Case 5

Anatomy & Embryology

History

A 36-year-old man complains of headaches and visual disturbances that began a few weeks ago and have been slowly getting worse. The patient says his peripheral vision seems to be decreased, but he denies double or blurry vision. The headaches are dull and generalized and seem to be worse in the morning. The patient denies fever, neck stiffness, cognitive deficits, or weakness. He last felt well 1 or 2 months ago and has no significant past medical history. The patient takes no medications and does not smoke or drink alcohol. Family history is unremarkable.

Physical Exam

The patient is in no acute distress. Eye exam reveals intact extraocular movements, but the patient has severe lateral visual field deficits in both eyes. Pupils are symmetric and react normally to accommodation and light. On chest exam, you note a bilateral clear nipple discharge, which the patient says began a few months ago. Abdominal and musculoskeletal exams are normal. No other neurologic deficits are detected.

Tests

Hemoglobin: normal
White blood cell count: normal
Prolactin level: markedly elevated

Questions

- What do you think is causing the patient's symptoms and signs?
- How would you describe the patient's visual deficit?
- Can you name some other types of visual field deficits and the location of lesions that cause them?

Bitemporal hemianopia (or hemianopsia) from a pituitary prolactinoma

Visual Pathways, Lesions, and Resulting Deficits

VISUAL FIELD DEFECT	LOCATION OF LESION
Right anopsia (monocular blindness)	Right optic nerve
Bitemporal hemianopsia	Optic chiasm (classically due to a pituitary tumor)
Left homonymous hemianopsia	Right optic tract
Left upper quadrant anopsia	Right optic radiations in the right temporal lobe
Left lower quadrant anopsia	Right optic radiations in the right parietal lobe
Left homonymous hemianopia with macular sparing	Right occipital lobe (from posterior cerebral artery occlusion)

Discussion

Bitemporal hemianopsia is the classic clinical visual pathway lesion, often caused by a pituitary adenoma, which may or may not secrete hormones. Things we see cross to the opposite side of the retina (e.g., the lateral visual field projects onto the medial or nasal aspect of the retina). The *medial retinal fibers decussate at the optic chiasm,* whereas the lateral retinal nerve fibers do not, explaining why both lateral visual fields are affected by a lesion of the optic chiasm, whereas a homonymous hemianopia can result from lesions of the optic tract.

Findings

Pituitary tumors classically have endocrine manifestations on the boards. The common type of hormonally active pituitary adenoma is the **prolactinoma,** which may cause a *bilateral, clear or milky nipple discharge* and menstrual irregularity in women. Other adenomas may secrete thyroid-stimulating hormone, growth hormone, or adrenocorticotropic hormone with resultant endocrine effects. Pituitary tumors also can cause local mass effect, such as *headaches* or **papilledema** (optic disc swelling from increased intracranial pressure).

Diagnosis & Treatment

Elevated pituitary hormonal levels are highly suggestive in the appropriate clinical setting. *MRI* is the preferred test to clinch the diagnosis. For smaller prolactinomas, **bromocriptine** can be given for treatment because it is a dopamine receptor agonist, and *dopamine inhibits prolactin secretion*. Larger tumors generally are surgically resected.

More High-Yield Facts

Antidiuretic hormone and **oxytocin** are secreted by the posterior lobe of the pituitary, but all other pituitary hormones are made by the anterior lobe.

Case 6

Anatomy & Embryology

History

A pregnant 25-year-old woman comes to the hospital while in labor. The woman, who is 36 weeks pregnant, has had no prior complaints and had a normal pregnancy. This is her first pregnancy. She has no significant past medical history, takes no medications, and does not smoke or drink alcohol.

Physical Exam

The exam is normal, and you can hear a normal fetal heartbeat with your stethoscope. The infant delivers vaginally without difficulty, and the umbilical cord is clamped. The infant appears healthy at birth.

Questions

- Describe the fetal circulation by naming the blood vessels, in order, that a fetal red blood cell (RBC) would travel through beginning at the point where the RBC picks up maternal oxygen at the placenta and ending at the point where the RBC returns to the placenta to release CO_2 and wastes.
- What are the three main fetal "shunts" in utero that facilitate getting oxygenated maternal blood to the fetus' systemic circulation?
- What happens to the fetal circulation after birth?
- Name the vessels (arteries or veins) that contain the blood with the highest oxygen saturation in the fetal circulation. How about after birth?

Topic Fetal circulation

Discussion

The fetal circulation is significantly different from that of the adult because the fetus gets oxygen from its mother, via the *placenta,* instead of through the lungs (i.e., the placenta provides respiratory function). Three primary shunts are designed to get the most oxygenated blood to the developing tissues: the **ductus venosus, foramen ovale,** and **ductus arteriosus.**

Anatomy

In utero, oxygen is released from maternal RBCs and picked up by fetal RBCs, which contain large amounts of fetal hemoglobin (e.g., *hemoglobin F*) and have an oxygen dissociation curve that is **shifted up and to the left** (i.e., greater oxygen affinity). This occurs in the **left umbilical vein,** the location of the blood with the highest oxygen saturation. Blood flows through the umbilical vein up to the liver, where most of it is shunted through the ductus venosus, bypassing the liver, to enter the inferior vena cava. From the inferior vena cava, blood flows into the right atrium, mixing with deoxygenated blood returning to the heart from the superior vena cava. Then the blood is largely shunted across the foramen ovale and into the left atrium, left ventricle, aorta, and systemic arteries to supply oxygen and nutrients to the developing organs.

When blood flows through the capillaries and returns to the heart by systemic veins, it goes into the right atrium and right ventricle and out into the main pulmonary artery. The pulmonary artery pressures are *high* because the lungs are not inflated, however, and most blood is preferentially shunted through the ductus arteriosus into the descending thoracic aorta. Blood returns to the placenta via the aorta and iliac arteries, then through the **umbilical arteries** to reach the placenta.

More High-Yield Facts

The left umbilical vein becomes the **ligamentum teres** (round ligament), and the umbilical arteries become the *medial umbilical folds;* the ductus venosum and arteriosum become their respective ligamenta.

After birth, the infant begins to breathe, decreasing pulmonary artery pressures, and the umbilical cord is clamped, stopping flow in the umbilical arteries and vein. Functional closure of the foramen ovale occurs as a result of decreased pulmonary resistance and increased left-sided heart pressures, and flow ceases through the ductus venosus. The ductus arteriosus also normally begins to close shortly after birth. When these changes have occurred, an adult circulation pattern is established, and the highest blood oxygenation levels are in the **pulmonary veins,** followed by the systemic arteries.

Case 7

Anatomy & Embryology

History

A 24-year-old man comes into the emergency department complaining of pain after a fall onto his outstretched right hand. The patient has no complaints besides right hand pain, is otherwise healthy, and takes no medications. His past medical history is unremarkable.

Physical Exam

When examining the right hand, you note that the patient has pain and deep tenderness in the anatomical snuff-box. Motor function and sensation are intact, and the rest of the exam is unremarkable.

Tests

Complete blood count: normal
X-ray of a normal right hand (not the patient's): see figure

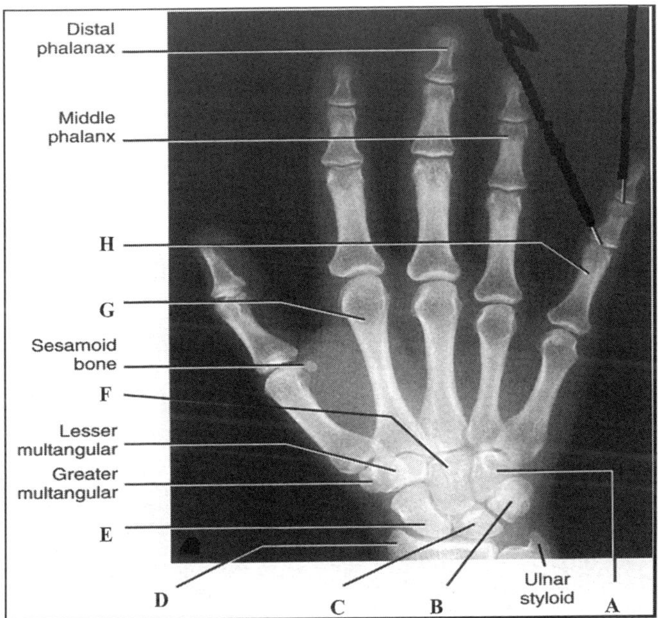

Questions

- Name the bones labeled *A* through *H* on the x-ray.
- What and where is the anatomical snuff-box?
- The given history and physical exam findings suggest a fracture to which bone?

Bones of the hand and wrist

Discussion

The radius (labeled *D* in the x-ray) and ulna articulate with the proximal row of carpal bones, forming the wrist joint. The distal row of carpal bones articulates with the metacarpal bones (*G* is the second metacarpal). The metacarpals articulate with the proximal phalanges (*H* is the fifth proximal phalanx) through the *metacarpophalangeal joints*. The *proximal interphalangeal joints* connect the proximal and middle phalanges, and the *distal interphalangeal joints* connect the middle and distal phalanges.

Many mnemonics have been developed to remember the location of the carpal bones (e.g., "*S*ome *l*overs *t*ry *p*ositions *t*hat *t*hey *c*an't *h*andle" covers the first letter of each of the carpal bones discussed in order). In the proximal carpal row (closer to the radius and ulna), the **scaphoid** (*E*) bone, which is also known as the **navicular,** begins the row on the thumb side of the wrist. Moving toward the ulna along the proximal carpal row, one finds the **lunate** (*C*) and the **triquetrum** (*B*) and **pisiform** bones, which are superimposed on each other on the x-ray.

In the distal carpal row, starting on the thumb side, one first sees the **trapezium** (also known as the greater multangular), and next to it the **trapezoid** (also known as the lesser multangular). Next comes the **capitate** (*F*), and last is the **hamate** bone (*A*).

The anatomical snuff-box is an area of skin depression on the lateral (i.e., thumb or radius side) aspect of the wrist just distal to the styloid process of the radius. Its boundaries are the tendon of the extensor pollicis longus medially and the tendons of the abductor pollicis longus and extensor pollicis brevis laterally. The **radial artery** pulse can be felt in this depression, and the scaphoid bone lies beneath the floor of the snuff-box, which is formed by the styloid process of the radius and the proximal aspect of the first metacarpal bone.

More High-Yield Facts

In a younger adult, pain and tenderness over the anatomical snuff-box after a fall on an outstretched hand should make you think of a *scaphoid (i.e., navicular) fracture,* which is what the patient in this case had.

Osteoarthritis generally affects the distal interphalangeal and proximal interphalangeal joints, whereas *rheumatoid arthritis* affects the more proximal metacarpophalangeal joints.

Case 8

Anatomy & Embryology

History

A 44-year-old woman comes into the office with a chief complaint of pain, numbness, tingling, and clumsiness in her right hand. She says the symptoms began a few months ago and have been getting worse, to the point where they are starting to interfere with her work as a typist.

The patient has strong and sometimes painful tingling sensations in the thumb, index, and middle fingers and the lateral (radial) side of her palm, which she says make her feel as though her hands have "fallen asleep." The woman also experiences numbness in the same areas. At times, the patient has dropped items she was holding in her hand because of hand weakness and clumsiness. The woman's past medical history is unremarkable. She takes no medications and has not been sexually active in the last few years. Family history is unremarkable.

Physical Exam

The patient is fit and healthy appearing. Head, neck, chest, abdomen, and lower extremity exams are normal. The patient has sensory loss in the thumb and first two and a half fingers of her right hand. Some thenar muscle atrophy and weakness also is noted in the right hand. Percussion of the volar (palmar) aspect of the distal right wrist reproduces the patient's typical tingling symptoms. The remainder of the exam is unremarkable.

Tests

Hemoglobin: 15 g/dL (normal 12–16 g/dL)
White blood cell count: 7800/μL (normal 4500–11,000/μL)
Platelet count: 280,000/μL (normal 150,000–400,000/μL)
Glucose: 92 mg/dL (normal fasting 70–110 mg/dL)
Creatinine: 0.9 mg/dL (normal 0.6–1.4 mg/dL)
Erythrocyte sedimentation rate: 8 mm/h (normal 0–20 mm/h)
Thyroid-stimulating hormone: 2.6 μU/mL (normal 0.5–5 μU/mL)
Urinalysis: normal

Question

- Damage to what nerve is causing the patient's neurologic symptoms?

Topic

Carpal tunnel syndrome (CTS) with median nerve compression

Discussion

The median nerve is supplied by nerve roots C5–T1 and crosses the wrist underneath the **flexor retinaculum** (along with the flexor digitorum, flexor pollicis longus, and flexor carpi radialis tendons). Clinically, it is commonly compressed here owing to various factors (e.g., trauma, arthritis, acromegaly), resulting in CTS.

The median nerve supplies sensation to the *lateral aspect (i.e., thumb side) of the palm* and the *palmar aspect of the thumb, index finger, and middle finger (and half the ring finger).* The median nerve also supplies motor fibers to the **thenar muscles** and lateral two lumbricals of the hand. In the forearm, the median nerve supplies the **pronator muscles** and all the **flexor muscles** except the **flexor carpi ulnaris** and the ulnar half of the flexor digitorum profundus (both supplied by the ulnar nerve).

Findings

Patients with CTS have **pain, tingling (paresthesia), or numbness** in one or both hands, in a median nerve distribution. In severe cases, *hypothenar muscle atrophy and weakness* may be present. Many patients report a history of repetitive forceful wrist flexion (e.g., occupational injury). **Hypothyroidism** and **acromegaly** are classic systemic causes, often resulting in bilateral CTS symptoms.

Treatment

Aspirin and other anti-inflammatory medications may help relieve symptoms. Surgery can be used to relieve pressure on the nerve if nonsurgical management fails.

More High-Yield Facts

The median nerve can be injured more proximally by a fracture of the humerus (supracondylar fracture). The resulting muscle denervation can cause *loss of the ability to pronate the forearm,* inability to flex the thumb, loss of opposition of the thumb, and weakened wrist flexion. *Flattening of the thenar eminence* also can occur, and the characteristic appearance has been called an "ape hand."

Compression or injury to the median nerve can lead to abnormally *slowed conduction velocity,* measured with a commonly used clinical test called a *nerve conduction study.*

Case 9

Anatomy & Embryology

History

You are called to see two different patients in your office, both with symptoms in their left upper extremities from a car accident several months ago. Patient 1 had a midshaft fracture of the left humerus at the time of the accident, and patient 2 sustained a fracture of the medial epicondyle of the distal left humerus.

Physical Exam

Patient 1 has wristdrop with weakness of forearm, wrist, and hand extension. She also has weakness of abduction and adduction of the hand and sensory loss over the back (dorsal aspect) of the thumb, first two fingers, and lateral hand (area *C* in the figure).

Patient 2 has a clawhand, with hyperextension of the fourth and fifth fingers at the metacarpophalangeal joints and flexion at the interphalangeal joints. He also has weakness of finger abduction and adduction and loss of thumb adduction and sensory loss over the area labeled *A* in the figure.

Tests

Hemoglobin: normal
White blood cell count: normal

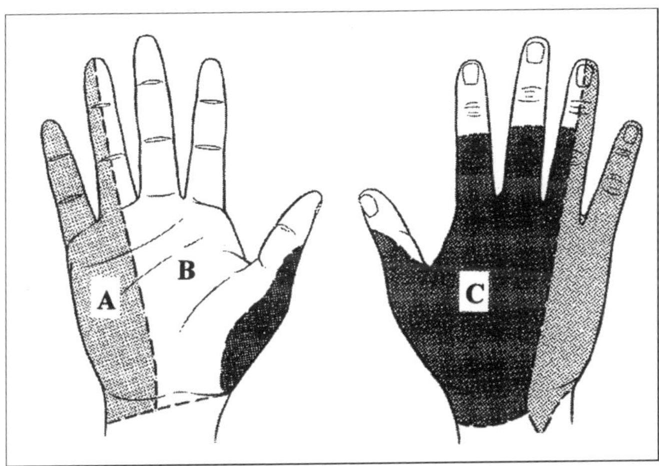

Questions

- What nerves are damaged in these two patients? What muscles do they supply?
- Which nerves supply cutaneous sensation to the areas labeled *A*, *B*, and *C* in the diagram?

Radial and ulnar nerves

Discussion

The three main nerves to the hand are the median, radial, and ulnar nerves. The radial and median nerves receive information from cord roots of levels **C5–T1,** whereas the ulnar nerve receives information from **C7–T1.** These are the three largest branches from the brachial plexus.

The radial nerve classically is injured by a **midshaft humeral fracture** or **pressure in the armpit** (e.g., caused by a crutch; a drunk who falls asleep with his arm hanging over the back of a chair). The ulnar nerve may be damaged by a fracture of the **medial epicondyle** of the distal humerus or penetrating trauma to the wrist.

Findings

Radial nerve damage (patient 1) can lead to weakness of the wrist extensors and **wristdrop** (wrist hangs limp owing to extensor weakness). Forearm, hand, metacarpal, and phalangeal extensors also are weakened, and patients develop *weakness of hand abduction and adduction.* Sensory deficits are shown in the figure (distribution *C*). The radial nerve also supplies the **triceps muscle.**

Ulnar nerve damage (patient 2) can cause **clawhand,** a characteristic appearance of the hand caused by *hyperextension of the fourth and fifth fingers at the metacarpophalangeal joints and flexion at the interphalangeal joints.* Damage also causes weakness of finger abduction and adduction, *loss of thumb adduction* (from adductor policis weakness), and sensory loss pattern *A* in the figure (*B* is the median nerve distribution). When you bump your elbow, you sometimes can "bump" your ulnar nerve—the sensation that results is why we call our elbow a "funny bone."

More High-Yield Facts

The axillary nerve supplies motor fibers to the **deltoid** and **teres minor** muscles and sensation to the lateral aspect of the arm (via the *lateral brachial cutaneous branch*).

The **lateral antebrachial cutaneous** nerve supplies sensation to the *lateral aspect of the forearm.* It arises from the **musculocutaneous nerve** (C5–C7), which also supplies motor fibers to the *coracobrachialis, biceps brachii, and brachialis muscles.*

The primary venous drainage from the hand and forearm is through the deep **brachial vein** and the superficial **basilic** (medial arm) and **cephalic** (lateral arm) veins. The brachial and basilic veins join to form the axillary vein, whereas the cephalic vein empties into the more proximal axillary vein.

Case 10

Anatomy & Embryology

History

A 44-year-old woman complains that her face looks "funny," especially when she smiles. The woman says her symptoms began a few weeks ago and have gotten worse. She mentions that everything sounds loud in her right ear, which started about the same time as her facial symptoms. The patient also mentions that she is unable to whistle, which she can usually do. The patient is fit and in no acute distress. She denies fever, headaches, sick contacts, and other neurologic symptoms. The patient has no significant past medical history; takes no medications; and does not use alcohol, tobacco, or drugs. Family history is unremarkable.

Physical Exam

You note flattening of the right nasolabial fold and a slight right facial droop. The patient is unable to close her right eye completely or wrinkle her right forehead. With smiling, an obvious asymmetry of the face is noted, as the right side of the patient's lips do not curl upward like the left side. On hearing testing, the patient is bothered by sounds in her right ear because they seem very loud to her. No sensory loss in the face is demonstrable. The remainder of the exam is unremarkable.

Tests

Hemoglobin: 15 g/dL (normal 12–16 g/dL)
White blood cell count: 7000/μL (normal 4500–11000/μL)
Platelet count: 280,000/μL (normal 150,000–400,000 μL)
Glucose: 92 mg/dL (normal fasting 70–110 mg/dL)
Creatinine: 0.9 mg/dL (normal 0.6–1.4 mg/dL)
Thyroid-stimulating hormone: 2.6 μU/mL (normal 0.5–5 μU/mL)
Urinalysis: normal
MRI of the brain: normal

Questions

- Damage to what cranial nerve is causing the patient's symptoms?
- Is it an upper or motor neuron lesion? How can you tell?
- What do you think the cause of the cranial nerve dysfunction is?

Topic Cranial nerve (CN) VII paralysis, in this case likely resulting from Bell's palsy

Discussion

CN VII arises from the *pons* and leaves the brainstem at the *cerebellopontine angle* to enter the *internal auditory meatus* (along with CN VIII), exiting the skull through the *stylomastoid foramen* of the temporal bone after passing through the facial canal. It contains afferent and efferent fibers. *General somatic afferent* fibers (**posterior auricular** branch, which relays sensation from the **skin of the external ear**) and *special visceral afferent* fibers (carry **taste from the anterior two thirds of the tongue**) have their cell bodies in the geniculate ganglion of the facial canal.

CN VII also contains *general visceral efferent* fibers, with cell bodies in the pterygopalatine and submandibular ganglia, which supply the **lacrimal, submandibular,** and **sublingual** glands (parotid supplied by CN IX). *Special visceral efferent* fibers supply the **muscles of facial expression,** and the **stylohyoid, stapedius,** and **posterior belly of the digastric** (CN V innervates the anterior belly) muscles.

Findings

"My face looks funny" and trouble eating (food collects between cheek and gum on affected side) and smiling are classic complaints in patients with a CN VII lesion. **Hyperacusis** (things sound louder on affected side owing to *stapedius muscle* paralysis) also can occur. The forehead muscles are *involved* with a lower motor neuron lesion (e.g., Bell's palsy), whereas they are typically *spared* in an upper motor neuron lesion (e.g., stroke, some brain tumors) because of dual innervation from upper motor neurons. The involved half of the face is *flat and expressionless.* A **facial droop; flattening of the nasolabial fold;** and **inability to whistle, wrinkle the forehead, or completely close the eye** on the affected side are typical findings with a lower motor neuron lesion. No significant sensory loss should be present with an isolated facial nerve lesion.

Causes of facial nerve paralysis are many and include Bell's palsy (classically considered idiopathic, though many cases may be due to latent **herpes simplex I** virus infection reactivation), stroke, tumor (classic is an **acoustic neuroma**/schwannoma in the cerebellopontine angle), *Lyme disease,* middle ear/mastoid infections, trauma, and multiple sclerosis.

More High-Yield Facts

CT or MRI of the brain helps rule out serious causes of CN VII lesion when there is *forehead sparing* on the affected side, *slowly progressive symptoms, or other neurologic findings* (e.g., CN VIII deficit).

Case 11

Anatomy & Embryology

History

A 45-year-old right-handed man complains of pain and weakness in his right shoulder. He thinks he may have injured his shoulder while throwing a ball back and forth with his son, but admits he had some pain in his shoulder before the throwing injury, which occurred 1 week ago. The patient says that his shoulder is weak when he tries to lift it from his side. The patient is otherwise healthy, has no known medical problems, and takes no regular medications. He works in construction, where he does a lot of lifting and heavy manual labor. The patient does not drink alcohol or smoke tobacco. Family history is notable for hypertension.

Physical Exam

Vital signs are normal. Neurologic exam is normal, and reflexes are normal in all four extremities. When comparing the two sides, you notice considerable weakness in the first 15° of abduction in the right shoulder compared with the left. If you passively lift the right shoulder into 15° of abduction, the patient has normal strength and ability to move the shoulder into greater degrees of abduction, although this action causes the patient to have pain in his shoulder. The rest of the exam is unremarkable.

Tests

Hemoglobin: 15 g/dL (normal 12–16 g/dL)
White blood cell count: 7800 µL (normal 4500–11,000/µL)
Erythrocyte sedimentation rate: 8 mm/h (normal 0–20 mm/h)

Questions

- What muscles make up the rotator cuff?
- Which of the four rotator cuff muscles arises anterior to the scapula?
- A tear in which rotator cuff muscle is likely the cause of this patient's symptoms?

Discussion

The patient in this case has a tear in the supraspinatus tendon, the most common cause of what is known as a "torn rotator cuff." The four muscles of the rotator cuff are the **supraspinatus, infraspinatus, teres minor**, and **subscapularis.** All arise from the scapula and insert into the humerus: the first three arise from the *posterior* aspect of the scapula and insert around the *greater* tuberosity; the subscapularis arises from the *anterior* aspect of the scapula and inserts around the *lesser* tuberosity.

The tone of the rotator cuff muscles assists in holding the head of the humerus in the fairly shallow glenoid cavity of the scapula. This provides stability to the shoulder, the *most commonly dislocated large joint in the body*. The major weakness of the rotator cuff is inferiorly, where no muscles exist. Dislocated shoulders generally lie inferior and anterior to the glenoid cavity (an "anterior" dislocation, which accounts for 90% to 95% of shoulder dislocations).

Although torn rotator cuffs are familiar to most professional baseball pitchers, they more commonly occur in *older individuals secondary to chronic degeneration* (i.e., "wear and tear"), often in people who perform repetitive shoulder movements (e.g., occupational). The supraspinatus is responsible for **the first 15 ° of shoulder abduction**, after which the *deltoid muscle* takes over and completes abduction to 90°. The infraspinatus and teres minor muscles help with lateral arm rotation, whereas the subscapularis helps rotate the arm medially.

Findings

The hallmarks of rotator cuff injury are **shoulder pain** and **limitation of shoulder movement;** later, disuse secondary to pain may lead to muscle *atrophy*. With supraspinatus injury or weakness, the most common clinical scenario, patients *cannot initiate abduction,* but can abduct 15° to 90° if the shoulder is passively abducted to 15°.

Treatment

Mild injury or strain can be treated with nonsteroidal anti-inflammatory drugs, whereas patients with a tendon tear (can be seen on MRI) usually are advised to have surgery.

More High-Yield Facts

The **quadrangular space** lies beneath the shoulder joint between the scapula and humerus. It is bounded superiorly by the teres minor, anteriorly by the inferior capsule of the shoulder joint and subscapularis, inferiorly by the teres major, laterally by the neck of the humerus, and medially by the long head of the triceps muscle. The **axillary nerve** (motor to deltoid and teres minor muscles and sensory to the skin over the lateral shoulder) and **posterior humeral circumflex** vessels course through this space. The axillary nerve may be damaged by a *fracture of the surgical neck of the humerus.*

Case 12

Anatomy & Embryology

History

A woman brings in her 1-month-old son for a routine visit. The infant was born without difficulty, is healthy and takes no medications. The mother reports no problems with the pregnancy. The infant is docile, and you note his increased neck tissue, oblique palpebral fissures, and prominent epicanthal folds while talking to the mother.

Physical Exam

The infant has multiple, small, circumferential, whitish spots on the periphery of the iris in each eye. The ears are small, and the nose is small with a flattened bridge. The infant keeps his mouth open, in part because of a protruding tongue. Diffuse mild muscle hypotonicity is present, and the infant has single palmar creases bilaterally. You note an abnormally wide gap between the first and second toes. Chest exam reveals clear lungs and a loud, harsh, holosystolic murmur heard best at the lower left sternal border.

Tests

Complete blood count: normal
Karyotype: see figure

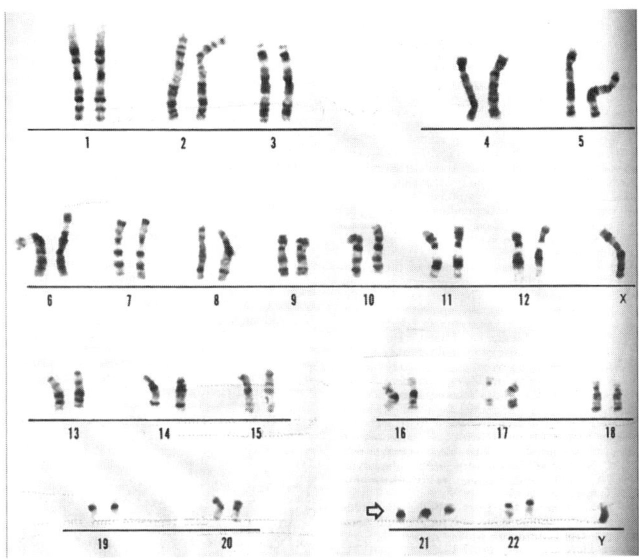

Questions

- What is the name of this patient's chromosomal abnormality (indicated by the *arrow* in the figure)?
- What are the two other classic trisomy syndromes?

Topic Down syndrome, or trisomy 21

Discussion

The karyotype reveals three copies of chromosome 21. In most cases of Down syndrome, there are three copies of chromosome 21, usually resulting from **maternal nondisjunction** during meiosis. Overall, the incidence is roughly 1/800, but the risk is increased with **increasing maternal age** so that the risk for 40-year-old mothers is 1/100, and the risk for 45-year-old mothers is 1/50.

Findings

Be able to recognize the clinical description of a case of Down syndrome. Classic features include **oblique up-slanting palpebral fissures,** prominent **epicanthal folds, Brushfield spots** (the white spots described on the iris), small nose with a **flat nasal bridge,** an **open mouth** with a **protruding tongue,** and increased neck tissue (**nuchal lymphedema,** which also can be seen in Turner syndrome). The hands are broad with a **single palmar crease** and incurvature of the **fifth finger (clinodactyly**). A wide **space between the first and second toes** is usually present.

Exam may reveal a murmur from a **congenital heart defect,** usually a **ventricular septal defect** or **atrioventricular canal defect.** Affected children are **mentally retarded** (average IQ roughly 50), they have an increased risk of **leukemia,** and most develop **Alzheimer's disease** by age 50.

Prevention

The child's **karyotype** should be obtained to determine if any genetic counseling is needed for the parents (e.g., if the child has a **translocation,** the risk of recurrence for the parents is higher and may be 100% with certain inherited translocations).

More High-Yield Facts

Trisomy 18 (Edward syndrome)—female predominance; look for microcephaly, **clenched fist with the index finger overlapping the third and fourth fingers** (almost pathognomonic), abnormal number of fingers (e.g., syndactyly, absent fingers), low-set ears, cleft lip/palate, short palpebral fissures, micrognathia, small mouth, nail hypoplasia, clubfeet, rocker-bottom feet, and cardiac malformations; mortality is 50% in the first 48 hours.

Trisomy 13 (Patau syndrome)—microcephaly, deafness, **holoprosencephaly** (brain not divided into two separate hemispheres); myelomeningocele, **microphthalmos,** low-set ears, cleft lip/palate, polydactyly, rocker-bottom feet, and cardiac anomalies; 70% die before 6 months of age.

Case 13

Anatomy & Embryology

History

A 44-year-old woman comes to the emergency department complaining of right upper quadrant abdominal pain. The woman has a history of gallstones and is obese.

Physical Exam

Exam shows low-grade fever and right upper quadrant tenderness in the region of the gallbladder. Acute cholecystitis is suspected, and the patient is taken to the operating room to have her gallbladder removed (cholecystectomy).

Surgery

The surgeon gains exposure to the gallbladder and biliary tree (see figure).

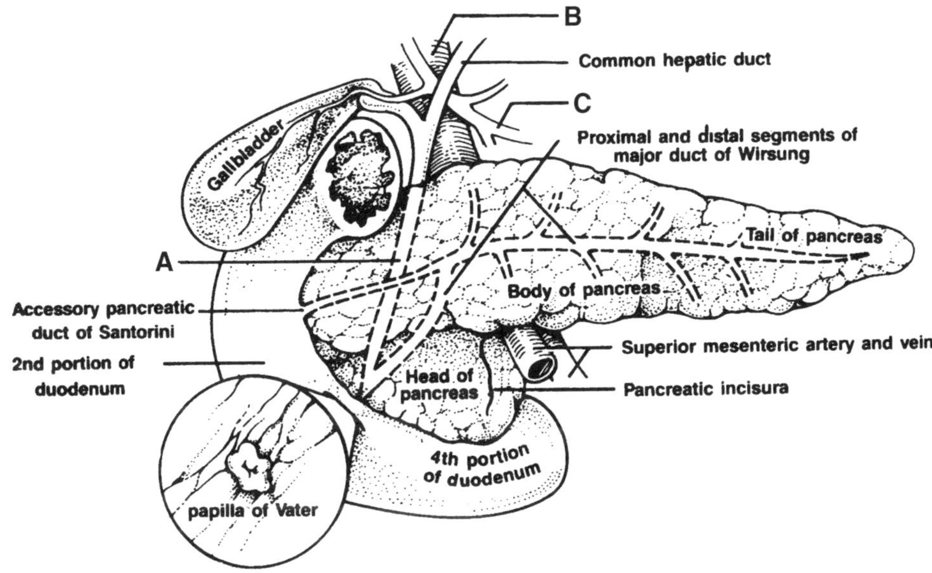

Questions

- Name the structures labeled *A, B,* and *C* on the figure.
- What is the porta hepatis? What is a portal triad?
- What is the relationship of the small branches of structures *A, B,* and *C* in the microscopic lobules of the liver (i.e., which is central and which is peripheral in a lobule)?

Porta hepatis

Discussion

The porta hepatis, or hilus of the liver, lies between the quadrate and caudate lobes on the underside (posteroinferior surface) of the liver and contains three primary structures: the **common bile duct** (CBD) (*A*), **portal vein** (*B*), and **hepatic artery** (*C*). The upper free edge of the lesser omentum is attached to the margins of the porta hepatis.

The anatomy of the porta hepatis becomes important when performing various types of gallbladder, biliary, liver, and duodenal surgery. The CBD and hepatic artery are *anterior* in relation to the portal vein; the CBD is more lateral than the artery (i.e., on the patient's right side).

The portal vein is formed behind the pancreatic head by the convergence of the *superior mesenteric and splenic veins* and supplies two thirds of the hepatic blood flow, bringing **products of digestion** from the intestine. The common hepatic artery is a branch of the *celiac trunk* (the other two celiac trunk branches are the splenic and left gastric) and provides **oxygen-rich** blood that makes up the other one third of hepatic flow. After giving off the gastroduodenal artery, the common hepatic is called the proper hepatic artery. The CBD forms from the right and left hepatic branches and receives the cystic duct, which leads to and drains the gallbladder. The CBD and the **major pancreatic duct of Wirsung** usually join and empty through a single conduit (emptying controlled in part by the *sphincter of Oddi*) into the second portion of the duodenum.

The tiny, polygonal classic **hepatic lobules** are the main functional parenchymal units of the liver. The smallest branches of the portal vein, CBD, and hepatic artery together are called **portal triads** and travel together in the *peripheral* aspect of a lobule. The smallest branches of the *hepatic veins* run through the *central* aspect of liver lobules, then form larger branches, and eventually empty into the inferior vena cava.

More High-Yield Facts

The macrophages of the liver are known as **Kupffer cells.** The liver is the second largest organ of the body (the *skin* is the largest).

The **Budd-Chiari syndrome** describes hepatic vein thrombosis. It usually is seen in association with *hypercoagulable states* (e.g., oral contraceptive use, malignancy, pregnancy).

Case 14

Anatomy & Embryology

History

A mother brings in her 4-year-old son at the request of his preschool teacher. The teacher claims, and the mother agrees, that the child is hyperactive and seems to have below-normal intelligence. The child's past medical history is notable for a ventricular septal defect, which was repaired shortly after birth, and the mother states that her son weighed only 6 lb (2725 g) at birth, although born at term. The mother states that the pregnancy was unremarkable. She has been battling alcoholism for the last 10 years, however, and admits to drinking during the pregnancy.

Physical Exam

The patient is active and responsive but seems to have delayed emotional and intellectual development, and you suspect mental retardation. Examination of the patient's face reveals maxillary and midface hypoplasia, shortened palpebral fissures, a flat nasal bridge, a thin upper lip, and a hypoplastic philtrum. The patient is restless and active during the exam and seems to be unable to hold still or pay attention for any significant amount of time. The remainder of the exam is unremarkable.

Tests

Hemoglobin: 12 g/dL (normal: 11–13 g/dL)
White blood cell count: 7000/μL (normal 4500–11,000/μL)
Creatinine: 0.9 mg/dL (normal 0.6–1.4 mg/dL)
Thyroid-stimulating hormone: 2.6 μU/mL (normal 0.5–5 μU/mL)
Urinalysis: normal
MRI of the brain: normal

Questions

- What is a teratogen? Which one is the likely cause for these findings?
- Can you name some other teratogens and the findings associated with them?

Topic Fetal alcohol syndrome (FAS)

Discussion

In the United States, FAS is the **most common cause of preventable mental retardation.** The threshold dose has not been established, so "**no alcohol is good alcohol**" during pregnancy. Other teratogens also may asked about on Step 1 (see table).

Severe cases typically occur in women who are heavy drinkers (>5 drinks/day). Children typically have **intrauterine growth retardation (IUGR),** are often born **small for gestational age,** and may have **microcephaly.** The pattern of poor growth may persist into early childhood.

Mental retardation, learning disorders/difficulties, and behavioral problems, including **attention-deficit hyperactivity disorder,** can be due to FAS. Motor skill and coordination may be impaired. Cardiovascular anomalies (classically **ventricular septal defect** or atrial septal defect) and skeletal, joint, and facial anomalies also can occur. The classic FAS facies are **short palpebral fissures, flat nasal bridge, maxillary and facial hypoplasia, a thin upper lip,** and a shortened philtrum (infranasal midline groove/depression of the upper lip).

More High-Yield Facts

Teratogens are agents that cause abnormal fetal development (e.g., birth defects). Examples are medications/drugs, infections, and radiation.

Common and/or Classic Teratogens

Agent	Anomalies Caused / Organ Systems Affected
Thalidomide	Phocomelia
Diphenylhydantoin	Craniofacial, limb, mental retardation, cardiovascular defects
Tetracycline	Yellow or brown teeth
Trimethadione	Craniofacial, mental retardation, cardiovascular defects
Aminoglycosides	Deafness
Diazepam	Cleft lip/palate
Warfarin	Craniofacial, IUGR, central nervous system, stillbirth
Valproic acid	Spina bifida, hypospadias
Isotretinoin	Central nervous system, craniofacial/ear, cardiovascular defects
Cigarettes	IUGR, low birth weight, prematurity
Cocaine	Cerebral infarcts, mental retardation, gastrointestinal, limb anomalies
Lithium	Cardiac anomalies (e.g., Ebstein's anomaly)
Diethylstilbestrol	Clear cell vaginal cancer, adenosis, cervical incompetence
Radiation	IUGR, central nervous system, facial anomalies, leukemia
Birth control pills	VACTERL syndrome (vertebral, anorectal, cardiac, tracheo-esophageal, renal and limb anomalies)

Case 15

Anatomy & Embryology

History

A 32-year-old man complains of an intermittent bulge in his right groin area that seems to get bigger when he coughs or strains. The patient first noticed his symptoms a few months ago, but the bulging now seems to be larger when it appears and occasionally causes a dull aching pain in his right lower abdomen and groin region. The patient is otherwise healthy, has no significant past medical history, and takes no medications. Family history is unremarkable.

Physical Exam

When the patient is in a standing position and coughs, you can feel a bulge enter his right scrotum from above. The bulge can be easily reduced manually. The area is nontender. The neck of the hernia sack seems to lie lateral to the inferior epigastric vessels and above and medial to the pubic tubercle.

Surgery

A surgeon takes the patient to the operating room and exposes the relevant anatomy. A schematic of the anatomy is shown in the figure.

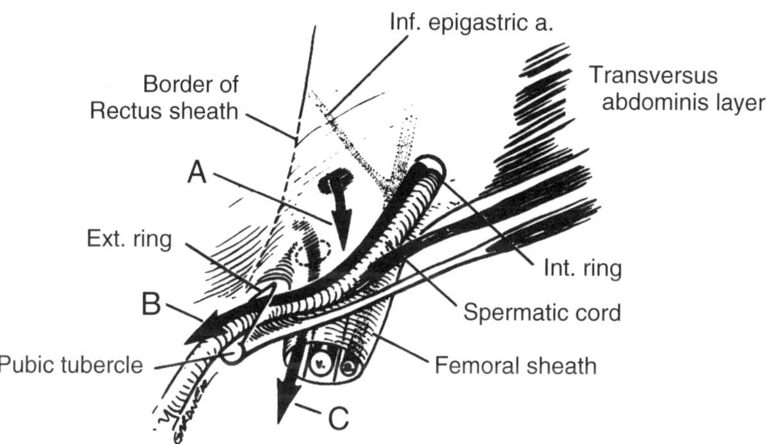

Questions

- Identify the three different types of groin hernias, labeled *A, B,* and *C* in the figure.
- Which type do you think the patient has? Which is the most common type?
- What forms Hesselbach's triangle, and which hernia type is it related to?

Inguinal canal

Discussion

The patient has an indirect inguinal hernia. The inguinal canals are passages through the lower anterior abdominal wall that transmit the spermatic cord in males (which contains the vas deferens, testicular artery and vein, and genital branch of the genitofemoral nerve), the round ligament in females, and the ilioinguinal nerve in both sexes. There are three types of groin hernias (hernias are protrusions of structures through the tissues that normally contain them): indirect (the most common), direct, and femoral.

Anatomy

The deep (or internal) inguinal ring is an opening in the transversalis fascia lateral to the inferior epigastric vessels and above the inguinal ligament. An **indirect hernia** (*B*) travels through this ring (i.e., *neck of hernia sac begins lateral to the inferior epigastric vessels*) and may exit through the superficial (or external) inguinal ring, a defect in the external oblique muscle. With a congenitally **patent processus vaginalis** (normally closes by birth), the hernia sac, which often contains small bowel within it, may travel down *into the scrotum or labia*. This type of hernia is more common in males and can occur at any age (classically in children and young adults).

A **direct inguinal hernia** (*A*) protrudes through a weakness in **Hesselbach's triangle**—the *neck of the hernia begins medial to the inferior epigastric vessels.* Hesselbach's triangle is defined superiorly and laterally by the inferior epigastric vessels, medially by the rectus abdominis muscle, and inferiorly by the inguinal ligament. The floor of the triangle is formed by the transversalis fascia. This type of hernia tends to be seen in older individuals. **Femoral hernias** (*C*) are more common in women and can be distinguished from inguinal hernias because *the sac of a femoral hernia lies below and lateral to the pubic tubercle* (versus above and medial to the tubercle for inguinal hernias).

Findings

The hernia bulge can be seen or felt (or both) on physical exam and by the patient. Be able to distinguish the type based on the location of the hernia neck or sac or both. Pain can occur from hernias, especially if the bowel gets trapped (**incarceration**) in the hernia sac, which may cut off the blood supply to the involved bowel (**strangulation**).

Treatment

Treatment is surgical repair.

More High-Yield Facts

The right gonadal (i.e., testicular or ovarian) vein drains into the **inferior vena cava,** whereas the left drains into the **left renal vein.**

Case 16

Anatomy & Embryology

History

You are asked to see a newborn infant who developed seizures starting 48 hours after birth. The infant began to have seizures and muscle spasms a few hours ago. He was born without complications but was noted to have a ventricular septal defect by physical exam shortly after birth, which was confirmed with cardiac ultrasound. There is no significant family history.

Physical Exam

The infant is lethargic, mildly tachypneic, and jittery, and you notice that he has severe carpopedal spasms. The infant has peculiar facies, with low-set ears, widely spaced eyes, and a small mandible. On chest exam, the lungs are clear bilaterally, but you note a 4/6 intensity, harsh holosystolic murmur along the lower left sternal border. There is a slight cyanotic tinge to the skin. Abdominal exam is unremarkable.

Tests

Complete blood count: normal
T-lymphocyte count: low
Renal and liver function tests: normal
Albumin: normal
Calcium: low
Chest x-ray: absent thymic shadow

Questions

- What congenital syndrome does this patient likely have?
- What are the adult derivatives of the embryologic branchial arches and clefts?
- What are the adult derivatives of the pharyngeal pouches? Which of these is related to this patient's condition?
- Are the pharyngeal pouches and branchial arches and clefts derived from ectoderm, mesoderm, endoderm, or the neural crest?

DiGeorge's syndrome

Discussion

DiGeorge's syndrome describes a failure of development of the third and fourth pharyngeal pouches, which leads to **hypocalcemia** (owing to the absence of parathyroid glands) and **immunodeficiency** (owing to absence of the thymus and resultant T-cell deficiency). Associated *facial and cardiac anomalies* are common, as described in the patient for this case.

The **pharyngeal pouches** are derived from **endoderm:**

Pouch	Adult Derivative
First	Middle ear cavity, eustachian tubes, tympanic membrane, mastoid air cells
Second	Epithelial lining of palatine tonsil
Third	Inferior parathyroids and thymus
Fourth	Superior parathyroids
Fifth	Ultimobranchial bodies (become calcitonin-secreting parafollicular/ C cells of thyroid)

The **branchial clefts** are derived from **ectoderm,** and each is associated with specific cartilaginous structures, muscles, and a cranial nerve:

Cleft	Adult derivative
First	External auditory meatus
Second through fourth	Temporary cervical sinuses (persistence leads to branchial cleft cysts in the neck)

The **branchial arches** are derived from **mesoderm** and **ectoderm,** are innervated by a cranial nerve, and form muscles and skeletal structures:

Arch	Cranial nerve	Cartilage and Muscle Derivatives
First	Trigeminal (V_3)	Meckel's cartilage (mandible, malleus, incus); muscles of mastication, mylohyoid, anterior belly of digastric, tensor tympani, and veli palatini
Second	Facial (VII)	Reichert's cartilage (stapes, styloid process, lesser horn of hyoid bone), muscles of facial expression, stylohyoid, posterior belly of digastric
Third	IX	Cartilage: greater horn of hyoid bone, stylopharyngeus muscle
Fourth through sixth	Vagus (X)	Cartilages: thyroid, cricoid, arytenoids, cuneiform; pharyngeal constrictor muscles, cricothyroid, and levator veli palatini (fourth arch); laryngeal muscles (sixth arch—recurrent laryngeal nerve)

More High-Yield Facts

Neural crest derivatives: sensory and autonomic ganglia, Schwann cells, melanocytes, pia and arachnoid layers of the meninges, adrenal medulla, odontoblasts, C cells of thyroid, and some enterochromaffin cells.

Case 17

Anatomy & Embryology

History

A 58-year-old woman complains of pelvic pain after an automobile accident. The patient was a restrained passenger in the front seat when the car she was in was hit by another vehicle at high speed. Her past medical history is unremarkable.

Physical Exam

The patient has some tenderness over the symphysis pubis, but the remainder of the exam is normal.

Tests

Complete blood count: normal
X-ray of the pelvis: see figure

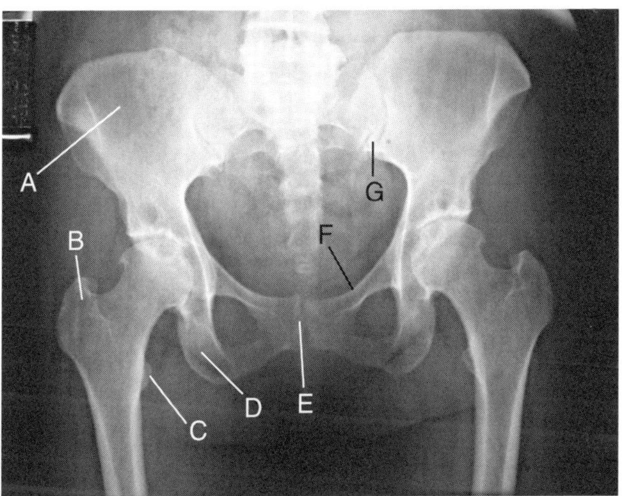

Questions

- Which of the labeled structures reflects the symphysis pubis?
- What is the name of the joint labeled *G* in the figure?
- Name the other labeled bony structures.
- What is the name of the structure that the femoral head articulates with to form the hip joint?

Topic Pelvic x-ray anatomy

Discussion

The bony pelvis comprises three major bones: the **ilium** (or iliac bone), **ischium,** and **pubis.** The iliac bone (labeled *A* in the figure) is the largest of the three, and its curved superior border is known as the *iliac crest,* an important anatomic landmark. The ischium (*D*) helps to support our weight when we sit down. The pubic bones (*F* labels the superior pubic ramus; below it lies the inferior pubic ramus) join in the midline at the **symphysis pubis** (*E*).

The three major pelvic bones all form part of the **acetabulum,** which is a shallow depression that articulates with the femoral head to form the hip joint. Two important bony protuberances arise from the femoral neck, where most hip fractures occur, at its junction with the femoral shaft: the **greater** (*B*) and **lesser** (*C*) **trochanters.** The gluteus medius and minimus, piriformis, and obturator internus muscles all insert onto the greater trochanter, whereas the iliopsoas muscle inserts onto the lesser trochanter.

Findings

The sacrum completes the bony pelvic ring and articulates with the iliac bones by the **sacroiliac joints** (*G*). These joints, along with the lower spine, classically are affected in **ankylosing spondylitis,** a seronegative (i.e., the serum is negative for rheumatoid factor) spondyloarthropathy (i.e., a disease that affects the vertebral joints). This condition can cause fusion of the sacroiliac joints and has a strong association with **HLA-B27** positivity.

More High-Yield Facts

There are four **hamstring muscles,** including the *biceps femoris, semitendinosus, semimembranosus,* and part of the *adductor magnus.* These muscles are located in the posterior fascial compartment of the thigh and act together to **extend the thigh** and **flex the knee.** These muscles are innervated by the **tibial nerve** (except the short head of the biceps femoris, which is supplied by the common peroneal nerve).

The **quadriceps** or quadriceps femoris muscle is a combination of four muscles that all converge to form a common quadriceps tendon, which inserts onto the patella, then extends by the ligamentum patellae to insert onto the tibial tubercle. The four muscles are the *rectus femoris, vastus lateralis, vastus medialis, and vastus intermedius,* which are located within the anterior fascial compartment of the thigh and act together to **extend the leg;** the rectus femoris also acts to flex the hip. These muscles all are supplied by the **femoral nerve.**

Case 18

Anatomy & Embryology

History

You are called to see a newborn infant for a growth on his back present at birth. The infant was delivered without difficulty several hours ago. The mother received no prenatal care but had no problems with the pregnancy. There is no signficant family history.

Physical Exam

The infant has an enlarged head. He actively moves both arms, but his legs are quite weak. Palpation of the lower spine reveals a defect in the area of the growth on the child's back. The child's appearance is shown in the figure.

Tests

Complete blood count: normal
Renal and liver function tests: normal
Ultrasound of the head: reveals dilation of the cerebral ventricles
X-ray of the lumbar spine: absent posterior elements of the spine from L2–S2.

Questions

- What term describes this infant's dilated cerebral ventricles?
- What is the general name of the disorder that encompasses this infant's condition?
- What happens if the anterior neuropore (i.e., cephalad end of the neural tube) fails to close or reopens during development? The posterior neuropore (i.e., caudal end of the neural tube)?
- What nutrient is associated with this infant's condition?

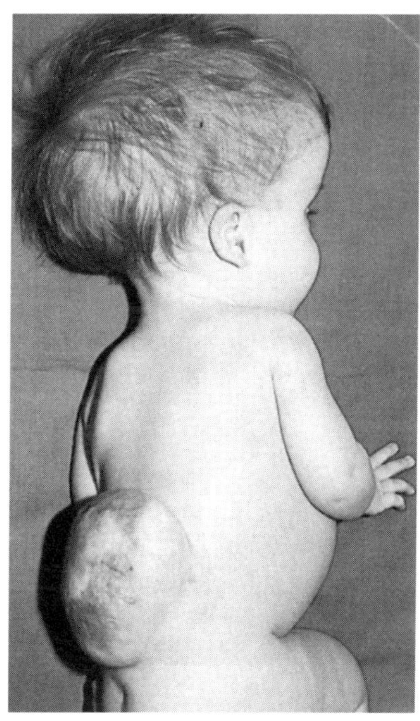

Topic Neural tube defects (NTDs)

Discussion

NTDs describe a spectrum of malformations affecting the central nervous system and supporting structures. The *neural tube* forms after the neural plate (**neuroectoderm**) develops neural folds, which fold around the neural groove to form a tube. The ends of the neural tube—the *anterior and posterior neuropores*—temporarily stay open to the amniotic cavity. The anterior neuropore normally closes first on day 23–25; the posterior neuropore typically closes on day 25 to 27.

Findings

Problems with neuropore closure account for most clinically seen NTDs, which include anencephaly, spina bifida, and other conditions. If the anterior (cephalad) neuropore fails to close, **anencephaly** may result. Anencephaly describes an *absence of the brain and cranial vault* (a rudimentary brainstem is usually present) and is uniformly fatal, usually in the first few days of life.

Failure of posterior (caudal) neuropore closure leads to **spina bifida,** which ranges in severity from mild (*spina bifida occulta,* a mild failure of posterior spine fusion that is associated with a **tuft of hair on the lower back**) to severe (*myelomeningocele* or myelocele). Most cases occur in the lumbosacral region of the spine, and more severe cases are associated with signficant neurologic deficits.

Prevention

Folic acid plays a role in the development of NTDs; reproductive-age women who take supplements have a greatly reduced risk of having children with NTDs should they become pregnant. Folic acid is recommended for all women who may get pregnant because neuropore closure happens early in utero, before many women know they are pregnant.

More High-Yield Facts

The **Arnold-Chiari malformation** (type II Chiari defect), which is what the child in this case had, typically includes a lumbosacral myelomeningocele, *small* posterior fossa with cerebellar tonsil herniation through the foramen magnum, and hydrocephalus (i.e., dilated cerebral ventricles, as in this patient).

The **Dandy-Walker malformation** describes an *enlarged* posterior fossa with absent cerebellar vermis and marked dilation of the fourth ventricle and hydrocephalus from atresia of the outlet foramina of **Luschka** and **Magendie.**

Case 19

Anatomy & Embryology

History

A 27-year-old woman who is 32 weeks pregnant comes into the emergency department while in labor. The infant is born as a stillbirth (not alive at the time of delivery).

This was to be the woman's second child, and she had no problems with her first pregnancy or her current one until a few hours ago, although the woman had no prenatal care. The woman does not smoke or drink alcohol and has no significant past medical or family history. Her other child is healthy. The woman wants to know why her infant was a stillborn.

Physical Exam

An autopsy is performed at the mother's request. The newborn's body is swollen and jaundiced. There are yellow bilirubin deposits noted in several areas of the brain, most prominent in the basal ganglia, and high bilirubin levels in the blood. The infant also is noted to have ascites and anemia.

Tests

Mother's blood type: O negative
Father's blood type: O positive
Infant's blood type: O positive

Questions

- What do the terms *positive* and *negative* mean when referring to blood type?
- What immunologic condition likely accounts for what happened to this patient and her infant?
- Are the parent's blood types relevant in this case? Why or why not?
- What do the terms *fetal hydrops* (i.e., hydrops fetalis) and *kernicterus* mean?

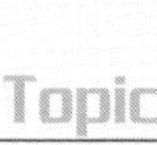

Rhesus (Rh) factor incompatibility and hemolytic disease of the newborn (also known as *erythroblastosis fetalis*)

Discussion

The Rhesus antigen in blood typing is second in importance only to the primary O-A-B system. There are six common types of Rh antigens, each of which is called an *Rh factor*. In practice, the presence or absence of the **D antigen** is most important because it is the most antigenic (i.e., most likely to cause an immune response or transfusion reaction). People are said to be *positive* (Rh+) if the D antigen is present on their blood cells and *negative* (Rh−) if not.

Findings

In the United States, 15% of whites and 8% of blacks are Rh−. If a woman who is Rh− is exposed to Rh+ blood (from prior fetal blood exposure or blood transfusion), she may form antibodies against the Rh antigen. IgG anti-Rh antibodies can cross the placenta and cause **hemolysis, anemia, hyperbilirubinemia,** and death (**fetal hydrops**) in an Rh+ fetus. Fetal hyperbilirubinemia, if severe, can lead to **kernicterus,** which describes bilirubin deposits in the brain that can lead to brain damage.

The mother has to be **Rh−** and the father has to be **Rh+** (or the father's blood type unknown) for the fetus to have a chance of being **Rh+**. Because a first exposure is needed to produce "sensitization" (i.e., a strong enough immune response to be clinically important), the *first pregnancy is often not affected,* but without prophylactic treatment, future pregnancies may develop serious complications. Other blood cell antigens (e.g., the **Kell** antigen) also can rarely cause a similar maternal-fetal incompatibility problem.

Prevention

Rh immune globulin (RhoGAM) is given routinely to Rh− pregnant women if the father's blood type is Rh+ to prevent sensitization before it can develop. RhoGAM attaches to the Rh antigen of fetal red blood cells that may be in the maternal bloodstream and prevents a maternal immune response by covering up the antigen. In current practice, potential cases of Rh incompatibility can be identified with routine screening of Rh status at a pregnant woman's first prenatal visit. Giving RhoGAM to prevent a future case (i.e., in the second pregnancy) of hemolytic disease of the newborn is an example of **primary prevention.**

More High-Yield Facts

An **indirect Coombs' test** can be ordered to detect the presence of Rh antibodies in pregnant women that are Rh negative.

Only **IgG** antibodies cross the placenta.

Case 20

Anatomy & Embryology

History

A 52-year-old man with known alcoholism, cirrhosis, and chronic hepatitis B comes in vomiting up blood. The patient has a long history of cirrhosis, jaundice, and abdominal distention. He takes no medications and does not smoke. Family history is notable for alcoholism. The patient denies fever or recent travel.

Physical Exam

The patient is jaundiced and has fresh red blood around his lips. Abdominal exam reveals abdominal distention with no masses. You note bulging flanks and a dull percussion note. An endoscope is passed through the patient's mouth and into his esophagus to examine the inside of the esophagus directly. Swollen, dilated veins can be seen under the mucosa of the esophagus.

Tests

Hemoglobin: low
Bilirubin: high
Schematic of the patient's portal venous system: see figure

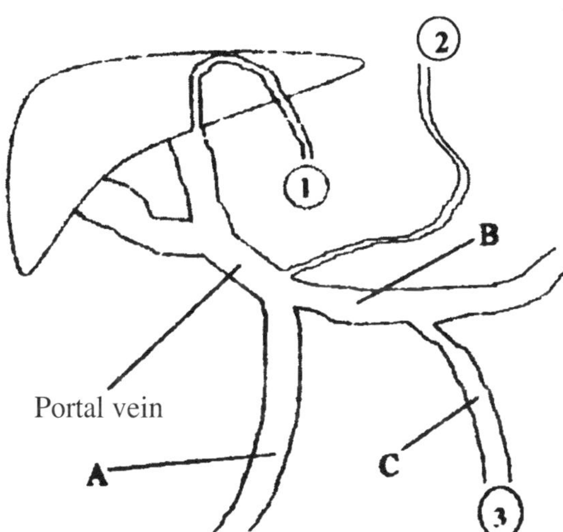

Questions

- What is the name of the condition seen with the endoscope? Why do these dilated veins develop?
- Name the venous structures labeled *A* through *C*.
- Name the portosystemic anastomoses that stem from the structures labeled *1* through *3* and their potential clinical consequences in cirrhosis.

Portal hypertension

Discussion

The portal vein is formed by the confluence of the *superior mesenteric vein* (*A* in the figure) and the *splenic vein* (*C*). The splenic vein receives the *inferior mesenteric vein* (*B*) before it joins the superior mesenteric vein. The *hepatic veins* drain the liver and empty into the inferior vena cava.

There are various *portosystemic anastomoses* that become significant only in pathologic states, especially portal hypertension, which most often is due to cirrhosis. The increased portal venous pressure can reopen one or more of these anastomoses owing to reversal of normal portal blood flow, resulting in shunting of portal blood into the systemic veins, with potentially important clinical consequences.

Findings

This patient has **esophageal varices** (the dilated veins seen in the esophagus), which are due to a portosystemic anastomosis between the *left gastric vein* (labeled *2* in the figure) and *azygous vein*. These can rupture as a result of increased pressure and cause life-threatening upper gastrointestinal hemorrhage. There also is an anastomosis between the *paraumbilical vein* (contained in the falciform ligament and adjacent to the ligamentum teres) and *inferior epigastric veins* around the navel (*1*), which can lead to **caput medusa** (enlarged visible veins on the anterior abdominal wall).

The final anastomosis (*3* in the figure) is between the *superior rectal vein,* which normally drains into the inferior mesenteric vein, and the *middle and inferior rectal veins*, which normally drain into the iliac venous system. This anastomosis can lead to **internal hemorrhoids,** which can be a cause of lower gastrointestinal hemorrhage.

Treatment

Treatment of portal hypertension is difficult in most cases, but an artificially created shunt created between the portal and systemic veins may reduce portal venous pressure and prolong survival.

More High-Yield Facts

The patient's abdomen is distended as a result of **ascites,** which causes *bulging flanks* and *dullness to percussion.*

Jaundice is common with severe cirrhosis, when the liver is no longer able to metabolize bilirubin normally.

Case 21

Anatomy & Embryology

History

A 42-year-old man presents with low back pain that began 2 weeks ago. The patient says his back began to hurt shortly after doing heavy yard work. He denies any motor weakness or sensory loss. His past medical history is unremarkable.

Physical Exam

The patient has a slightly limited range of motion in the lower back secondary to pain, and you notice some mild muscle spasm in the muscles of the lower back. The rest of the exam is unremarkable

Tests

Complete blood count: normal
Schematic of a lumbar vertebra and the lumbar spine ligaments: see figure

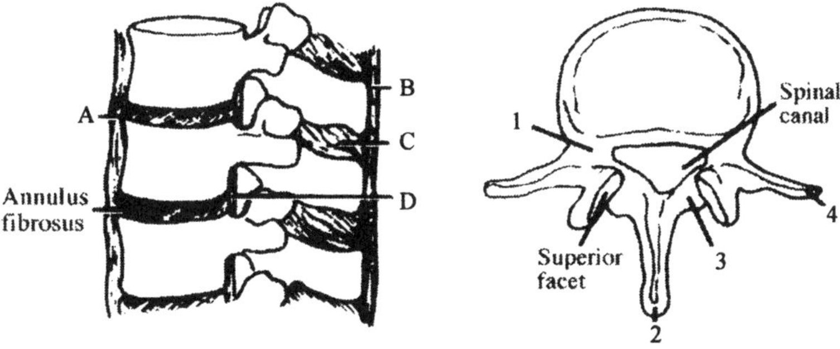

Questions

- Name the spinal ligaments labeled *A* through *D* and the lumbar vertebrae parts labeled *1* through *4* in the figure.
- How many cervical, thoracic, and lumbar vertebrae are there?
- At what lumbar level does the spinal cord terminate in the adult? The young child?
- From what artery does the anterior spinal artery arise?

Discussion

The spinal column is made up of *7 cervical, 12 thoracic, and 5 lumbar vertebrae.* There are some differences in the vertebral bodies at the different levels. The cervical vertebrae contain transverse foramina within their transverse processes, through which pass the vertebral arteries. The thoracic vertebrae contain costal facets that articulate with the ribs, and the vertebral bodies get bigger as one moves inferiorly.

Anatomy

The schematic of the lumbar spine ligaments also applies to the thoracic and cervical spine. The **anterior longitudinal ligament** (labeled *A* in the figure) runs along the anterior surface of the vertebral bodies. The **posterior longitudinal ligament** (*D*) runs along the posterior surface of the vertebral bodies, at the anterior boundary of the spinal canal.

The **ligamentum flavum** (not shown) runs along the posterior boundary of the spinal canal against the anterior surfaces of the lamina (a left lamina is labeled *3* in the figure). Running between the spinous processes are the **interspinous ligaments** (*C*). Connecting the tips of the spinous processes is the **supraspinous ligment** (*B*), which lies posterior to the interspinous ligaments.

Each vertebral body is composed of an anterior vertebral body and a posterior *vertebral arch,* with the exception of the atlas (C1), which is a complete ring with no body (the dens of C2 acts as its specialized body). The vertebral arch is made up of paired **pedicles** (*1*) anteriorly, which connect to the paired **laminae** (*3*) posteriorly. Where the pedicles join with the laminae, bony *transverse processes* (*4*) extend laterally, and where the two laminae meet, the *spinous process* (*2*) extends posteriorly.

More High-Yield Facts

In a young child, the spinal cord terminates at about the level of the **L2–L3** interspace. As the child grows, the spinal cord comes to lie at the **inferior aspect of L1,** terminating in the tapered *conus medullaris*. The *filum terminale* is a thickened prolongation of the pia mater that extends from the tip of the conus medullaris to the end of the dural sac (*S2*), where it continues as the external filum and inserts on the posterior coccyx.

The *anterior spinal artery* arises from both **vertebral arteries** and descends along the anterior aspect of the spinal cord to supply the *anterior two thirds* of the spinal cord.

Case 22

Anatomy & Embryology

History

A 74-year-old woman comes into your office several weeks after having a stroke for follow-up. The patient complains of trouble swallowing and hoarseness. She wonders if it might be due to her stroke. She has a history of hypertension and takes atenolol. Family history is significant for myocardial infarction in her mother and a stroke in her father.

Physical Exam

The extraocular movements are normal, the pupils are equal and normally reactive, and there are no visual field defects. Facial movements and sensation are intact. You notice that the patient has a hoarse voice, which she tells you began around the time of her stroke. The patient's gag reflex is absent, and she has trouble elevating her palate. Taste is intact in both the front and back of the tongue. The rest of the exam is normal.

Tests

Hemoglobin: normal
White blood cell count: normal
Electrolytes: normal

Questions

- What cranial nerve is likely accounting for the patient's symptoms and physical exam findings?
- What are the functions of this nerve (i.e., what does it innervate)?
- From what part of the brainstem does this nerve arise?
- A lesion to what cranial nerve would cause difficulty turning one's head to one side and shoulder droop? If a lesion to this nerve is on the right, what side would these clinical deficits be on?

Topic Vagus nerve (cranial nerve X)

Discussion

The fibers of the vagus nerve originate from four nuclei (the *solitary, dorsal motor,* and *ambiguus*) in the **medulla.** Cranial nerve X innervates structures from the meninges down to the abdomen, including the external ear, palate, pharynx, larynx, thoracic and abdominal viscera, and gastrointestinal tract from the esophagus to the splenic flexure of the colon (i.e., foregut and midgut).

General sensory afferent vagus fibers supply the external ear and meninges. *General visceral afferent* fibers supply the respiratory and gastrointestinal tracts and the aortic arch baroreceptors and chemoreceptors. *Special visceral afferent* fibers carry taste information from the posterior oral cavity (not the tongue), whereas *general visceral efferent* fibers supply the gut, respiratory structures, and heart. The striated muscles of the palate, pharynx, and larynx are supplied by *special visceral efferent* vagal fibers.

Findings

With a lesion of the vagus nerve, patients usually complain of **difficulty swallowing** (dysphagia) or **hoarseness** (if the recurrent laryngeal branch of the vagus is affected) or both. Patients have difficulty **elevating the palate** and **loss of the gag reflex** (the glossopharyngeal nerve is the *afferent* or sensory limb of this reflex, the vagus is the *efferent* or motor limb).

More High-Yield Facts

The **recurrent laryngeal** branch of the vagus on the right hooks around the right subclavian artery and ascends into the neck between the esophagus and trachea. On the left, this branch hooks around the *arch of the aorta adjacent to the ligamentum arteriosum,* then also ascends in the groove between the esophagus and the trachea.

In some patients with peptic ulcers, lesions are surgically created in the vagal fibers supplying the stomach to *reduce acid secretion.*

A lesion to cranial nerve XI (the spinal accessory nerve), which also arises from the medulla, causes paralysis of the **sternocleidomastoid** and **trapezius** muscles on the side of the lesion. The clinical result is **drooping of the shoulder** and mild winging of the scapula *on the side of the lesion* and **difficulty in turning the head** *to the side opposite the lesion.*

Case 23

Anatomy & Embryology

History

You are asked to examine an infant with a heart murmur. The infant was born prematurely to a mother who had a rubella infection early in the pregnancy.

Physical Exam

The infant is small but active and seems mildly short of breath. On auscultation of the chest, you hear a harsh, machine-like, continuous murmur in the upper left parasternal area. The rest of the exam is normal.

Tests

Hemoglobin: normal
Electrolytes: normal
Infant's cardiovascular structures: see figure

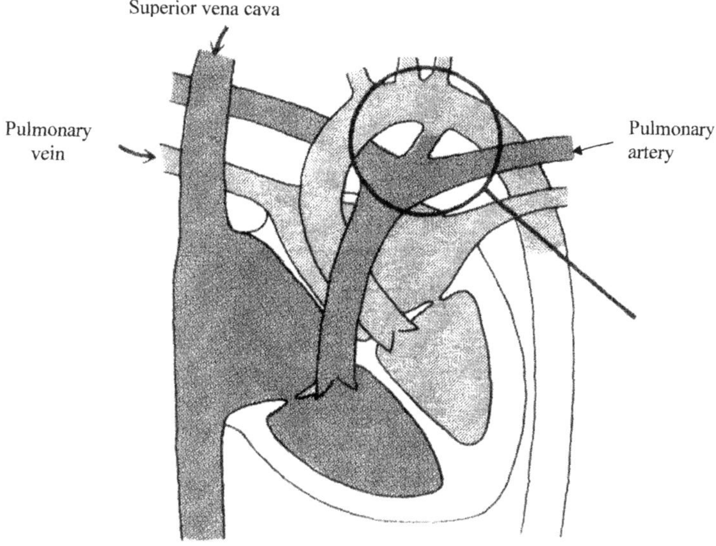

Questions

- What is the abnormal structure circled in the figure?
- What is its role in the circulation in utero? After birth?
- What physiologic conditions develop after birth that cause functional and anatomic closure of this structure?
- What drugs are given to affect this structure?

Patent ductus arteriosus (PDA)

Discussion

In utero, respiratory function is provided by the placenta, and the lungs are not needed to oxygenate the blood. The collapsed, developing lungs and low oxygen tension in the fetal circulation result in high pulmonary arterial resistance. In utero, aortic pressures are lower than pulmonary artery pressures. Blood from the right ventricle goes into the pulmonary artery and is preferentially routed through a special artery called the *ductus arteriosus,* which connects the pulmonary artery and aortic arch (just below the left subclavian artery origin).

At birth, infants' lungs inflate with air. This inflation results in reduced pulmonary vascular resistance and decreased pulmonary artery pressures. At the same time, blood flow through the placenta ceases, and systemic arterial blood pressure rises. The result is higher pressure in the aorta than the pulmonary arteries and subsequent temporary reversal of flow through the ductus arteriosus. The higher blood oxygen concentrations after birth are thought to cause smooth muscle constriction in the ductus (prostaglandin mediated), resulting in its closure within a few days in normal infants.

Findings

In some children, particularly preterm infants, the ductus may remain open and cause a left-to-right shunt, as high-pressure aortic blood flow is shunted through the ductus into the pulmonary circulation. This shunt results in increased pulmonary blood flow, which can compromise respiratory function and may lead to rapid breathing and congestive heart failure. On exam, there is a continuous, harsh, machine-like murmur heard best in the upper left parasternal region (second intercostal space).

Treatment

Prostaglandin-synthesis inhibitors (typically **indomethacin**) can be given in an attempt to close a PDA. These agents shut off production of prostaglandin E, a substance that causes vasodilation in the ductus. If indomethacin fails, **surgical ligation** of the PDA can be done. With certain complex congenital heart anomalies (e.g., tricuspid or pulmonic atresia), a PDA ironically must be intentionally maintained (to permit survival) with pharmacologic doses of **prostaglandin E_1** until surgery can be performed.

More High-Yield Facts

PDA has been associated with maternal (and resultant fetal) **rubella** infection during pregnancy.

In adults, the ductus arteriosus becomes the **ligamentum arteriosum.**

Case 24

Anatomy & Embryology

History

A 34-year-old man complains of altered sensation and weakness. The patient says he began to develop an increasingly severe decline in sensation in his shoulders and upper arms a few months ago, followed by weakness in these same muscle groups. The patient denies pain, fever, headache, trauma, seizures, weight loss, and night sweats. His past medical history and family history are unremarkable. The patient takes no medications, eats a healthy diet, and does not smoke or drink alcohol.

Physical Exam

You note loss of pain and temperature sensation over the back of the neck, upper back, shoulders and upper arms in a capelike distribution. Fine touch and vibration sense is preserved in these regions. Bilateral atrophy and weakness of the hand and distal arm muscles is noted, with associated diminished reflexes in these areas. The remainder of the exam is normal.

Tests

Hemoglobin: normal
Erythrocyte sedimentation rate: normal
Spinal cord lesions: see figure (dark gray areas)

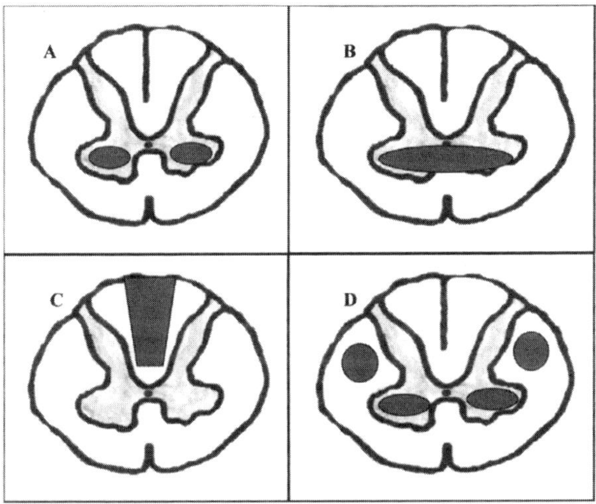

Questions

- Which of the lettered figures explains this patient's neurologic deficits? What is the condition responsible called?
- Match each of the remaining lettered figures with one of the following conditions: amyotrophic lateral sclerosis, dorsal column disease in tertiary syphilis, and poliomyelitis.

Syringomyelia

Discussion

Syringomyelia describes an abnormal, fluid-filled cavitation of the spinal cord. It can be idiopathic or due to developmental factors (e.g., associated with the Arnold-Chiari malformation), prior trauma, or tumors affecting the spinal cord. Cavitation often begins in the **central cervical spinal cord** *adjacent to the central canal,* gradually increasing in size.

Findings

A fairly specific order and distribution of neurologic symptoms classically occurs in syringomyelia, resulting from progressive involvement of different spinal cord tracts. Initially, there is destruction of the ventral white commissure and interruption of decussating spinothalamic tract fibers, which causes **bilateral loss of pain and temperature sensation in a capelike distribution,** as described in the case patient. *Motor weakness in the hands and arms* follows when the cavity extends into the ventral horns, affecting *lower motor neurons.*

Figure *A* shows bilateral ventral horn lesions, which would affect the anterior horn cells and cause lower motor neuron lesions, as in **poliomyelitis** or **Werdnig-Hoffman disease.** *C* depicts a lesion in the dorsal columns, as can occur in **syphilis (tabes dorsalis)** and **vitamin B_{12} deficiency.** *D* shows the lesions of **amyotrophic lateral sclerosis** (Lou Gehrig disease), with involvement of lower (ventral horns) *and* upper (lateral corticospinal tracts) motor neurons.

The **dorsal columns** carry sensory information from the ipsilateral side related to *tactile discrimination, position sense, and vibration.* This tract decussates in the caudal medulla (in the medial lemniscus), so cord lesions cause ipsilateral deficits. The **corticospinal tracts** decussate in the caudal medulla and travel laterally within the cord. Lesions in the cord produce ipsilateral upper motor neuron deficits, whereas lesions of this tract above the decussation (e.g., motor cortex stroke) cause contralateral deficits.

More High-Yeld Facts

Vitamin B_{12} deficiency, which most often occurs in the setting of pernicious anemia, can affect not only the dorsal columns, but also the spinocerebellar tracts and corticospinal tracts, resulting in ataxia (lack of coordination) and upper motor neuron deficits.

Case 25

Anatomy & Embryology

History

A 17-year-old boy of Mediterranean descent comes into the office needing a routine physical exam so that he can participate in athletics at school. The patient has no complaints and is in good health. He has no significant past medical history, takes no medications, and exercises regularly without difficulty. Family history is significant for anemia.

Physical Exam

The vital signs are normal. You note mild mucous membrane pallor, but the exam is otherwise unremarkable.

Tests

Hemoglobin: slightly low
White blood cell count: normal
Platelet count: normal
Hemoglobin electrophoresis:
Hemoglobin A_2: elevated
Hemoglobin F: elevated
Iron level: normal
Ferritin: normal
Peripheral blood smear: reveals microcytosis, hypochromia, and multiple cells that resemble "targets" (*arrows* in figure).

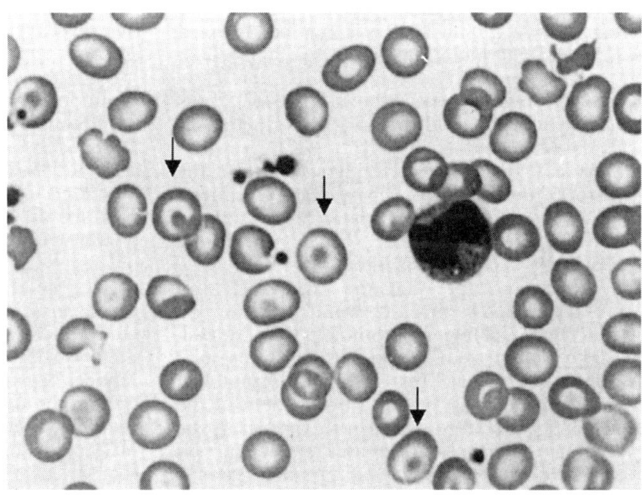

Questions

- What condition does this patient have?
- What population groups are commonly affected?

Topic Thalassemia

Discussion

This patient has β–thalassemia minor. The primary adult hemoglobin, *hemoglobin A,* contains two α-globin and two β-globin chains. There are four α-globin genes (two pairs), located on *chromosome 16.* There are only two β-globin genes, located on *chromosome 11.* Mutations in these genes can cause reduced or absent synthesis of the respective globin chain and a relative excess of the unaffected chain. Severity is related to the number of genes affected.

Decreased globin production leads to **hypochromic** (pale) red blood cells, whereas excess of the other chain leads to **ineffective erythropoiesis** and **peripheral hemolysis.** Clinical severity can range from asymptomatic to in utero death. Thalassemia is most common in people of **African, Mediterranean, Middle Eastern,** and **Asian** descent.

Findings

Patients affected with clinically significant α-thalassemia (three α genes deleted, called *hemoglobin H disease*) have abnormalities **at birth** (and in utero), because α chains make up fetal hemoglobin (hemoglobin F) and hemoglobin A_2, and all important forms of hemoglobin are affected. Patients with no normal copies of the α gene *die in utero* as a result of hypoxia **(hydrops fetalis**). Because however, there are four copies of the α gene, however, individuals with only one or two abnormal copies are able to make enough α globin chains to remain asymptomatic (*silent carriers* or *thalassemia trait*).

Patients with β-thalassemia are usually not symptomatic until **after 4 or 5 months of age** because of the presence of fetal hemoglobin at birth. One minor gene alteration is asymptomatic, but a totally defective β-globin gene (*thalassemia intermedia*) or two abnormal genes (*Cooley's anemia* or *β-thalassemia major*) cause significant, transfusion-requiring anemia.

Diagnosis & Treatment

The diagnosis of either thalassemia type can be made with **hemoglobin electrophoresis.** Bone marrow transplant can be curative in severe cases.

More High-Yield Facts

Asymptomatic adults with thalassemia have **microcytic, hypochromic red blood cells; target cells** (see figure, *arrows*); and usually an asymptomatic **mild anemia** that *can be confused with iron-deficiency anemia.* **Iron studies are normal** in individuals with thalassemia, however, distinguishing it from iron-deficiency anemia. In β-thalassemia minor, look for an **elevated hemoglobin A_2** or **elevated hemoglobin F,** which are *not* seen with α-thalassemia minor (because both contain α chains). *Do not give these patients iron* (may cause iron overload).

Case 26

Anatomy & Embryology

History

A 52-year-old man complains of low back pain that radiates into the right hip and lateral right thigh. He also says that his right leg is "clumsy" at times. The patient's symptoms started 1 month ago after doing some heavy lifting and have been intermittent but gradually worsening and more frequent. The patient has a history of obesity but has no other medical problems and takes no medications. He denies fever or weight loss. Family history is unremarkable.

Physical Exam

You note a decreased biceps femoris reflex on the right compared with the left. The patient also has weakness of foot and ankle dorsiflexion on the right. You also find sensory loss over the dorsal aspect of the right foot, including the medial toes and space between the great and second toes, and the lateral aspect of the right leg. A straight-leg raise test reproduces the patient's pain.

Tests

Hemoglobin: normal
White blood cell count: normal
MRI of the lumbar spine: see figure

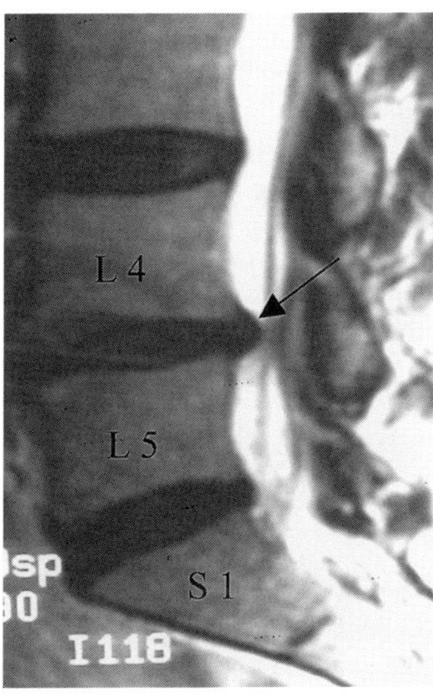

Questions

- What structure is the arrow in the MRI scan pointing to?
- What nerve root is affected by this patient's condition?
- Where does this condition most commonly occur?

Topic Herniated lumbar disc

Discussion

The *arrow* in the figure points to the L4–L5 intervertebral disc, which is bulging posteriorly (compare with other levels), resulting in the right L5 nerve root irritation this patient is experiencing. With age, degeneration of intervertebral discs can occur, with the potential for herniation of the central substance of the disc, called the **nucleus pulposus,** through a tear in its surrounding **annulus fibrosus.** This situation can result in back pain and spasm and neurologic symptoms related to irritation of adjacent nerve roots.

Disc herniation is usually in a posterolateral direction (although other directions can occur), which irritates the *next lower ipsilateral nerve root* (e.g., a herniated L4–L5 disc affects the ipsilateral L5 nerve root). The lower lumbar spine (i.e., L5–S1 and L4–L5 discs) is the most common location, followed by the lower cervical spine (C5–C6 and C6–C7).

Findings

Lesion Localization Based on Neurologic Deficits

Disc Level (Nerve Root)	Reflex / Motor	Sensory
L5–S1 (S1)	**Achilles reflex** **Plantar flexion**	Lateral foot and leg, hip, **lateral toes**
L4–L5 (L5)	Biceps femoris reflex (rare) **Ankle and foot dorsiflexion**	Dorsal foot, **medial toes,** web space between great and second toe, lateral thigh/leg
L3–L4 (L4)	**Patellar reflex** Quadriceps, gluteus medius	**Medial calf,** anterior lower thigh
C5–C6 (C6)	**Biceps reflex** Deltoid and biceps muscles	Thumb and index fingers
C6–C7 (C7)	**Triceps reflex** Triceps, forearm extensors	Index and middle fingers

The **straight-leg raise test** (patient lies on back and you raise the straightened leg off the table) usually reproduces/aggravates symptoms. A far lateral lumbar disc herniation (much less common) may affect a nerve root that is one level higher than expected (e.g., L4–L5 disc affects L4 root instead of L5).

Treatment

If conservative treatment (e.g., rest, physical therapy, pain relievers) fails, surgery may be needed.

More High-Yield Facts

A *lumbar puncture* is used to obtain cerebrospinal fluid for diagnostic purposes (e.g., suspected meningitis). A needle passed through the lower back traverses the following structures (in order) to reach the cerebrospinal fluid–containing subarachnoid space: skin, *superficial fascia, supraspinous ligament, interspinous ligament, ligamentum flavum, fatty tissue containing the vertebral venous plexus, dura mater, and arachnoid mater.*

Case 27

Anatomy & Embryology

History

A 76-year-old woman has severe abdominal pain that began a few hours ago and has been getting worse. The patient has a history of hypertension, severe atherosclerosis, and two prior myocardial infarctions. The patient takes multiple medications for hypertension and high cholesterol. Family history is significant for myocardial infarctions and strokes.

Physical Exam

After the physical exam, which reveals severe abdominal tenderness and decreased bowel sounds, you suspect ischemia to the bowel. You order angiography to evaluate the abdominal aorta and its branches.

Tests

Hemoglobin: low
White blood cell count: normal
Normal abdominal aorta seen at angiography: see figure

Questions

- What is the relationship between the aorta, inferior vena cava, and esophagus as they traverse the diaphragm (anterior to posterior and vertebral level)?
- What is the relationship of the abdominal aorta to the spine and the inferior vena cava?
- What are the major abdominal aorta trunks and branches labeled *A* through *E* in the figure? What embyologic gut segments are supplied by *A*, *B*, and *C*?
- What segment of bowel is prone to be damaged with gut ischemia because it lies within the "watershed" vascular territory between the distribution of the superior and inferior mesenteric arteries?

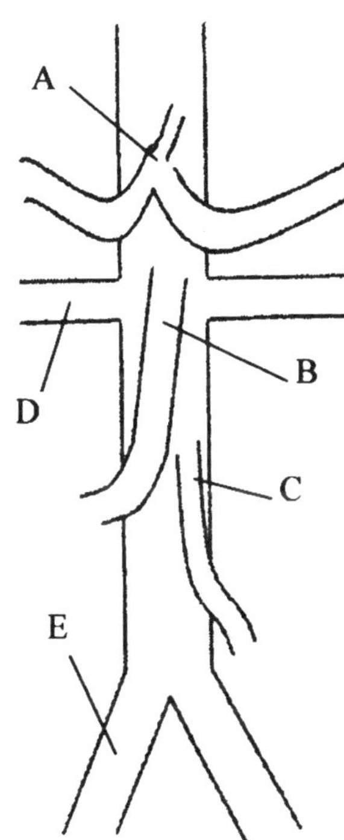

Abdominal aorta and its branches

Discussion

The descending thoracic aorta becomes the abdominal aorta as it passes through the aortic hiatus of the diaphragm with the **thoracic duct** and **azygos vein** at the level of *T12,* posterior to the esophagus and the inferior vena cava (vena cava most anterior of the three). The abdominal aorta lies anterior to the spine to the left of the midline and the inferior vena cava.

The embryologic **foregut** (*esophagus to duodenum, includes liver and pancreas*), **midgut** (*duodenum to splenic flexure* region of colon), and **hindgut** (*splenic flexure to rectum*) are supplied by the **celiac axis/trunk** (*A* in figure), **superior mesenteric artery** (*B*), and **inferior mesenteric artery** (*C*), respectively. Clots (e.g., from the heart in atrial fibrillation) can embolize into these branches (usually the superior mesenteric artery) and cause gut ischemia, or chronic ischemia can occur from atherosclerosis or hypoperfusion (e.g., hypotension).

Because the vascular territories of the superior and inferior mesenteric arteries stop in the region of the *splenic flexure of the colon* (junction of the transverse and descending colon), this segment is at risk for ischemia. A segment of anatomy in such a position is said to be in a *watershed* area (term also used in the brain for the border between the main cerebral artery territories).

Findings

Bowel ischemia, when severe, can lead to bowel *infarction,* a life-threatening problem (> 50% mortality). Infarcts are generally **hemorrhagic,** and patients may develop bloody diarrhea along with severe abdominal pain and tenderness. Affected bowel often must be resected surgically in an attempt to prevent bowel perforation, which can lead to *sepsis, shock, and death.*

More High-Yield Facts

The renal arteries (*D*) take off from the aorta between the origin of the mesenteric arteries. The aorta bifurcates into the **common iliac arteries** (*E*) at the level of L4.

The esophagus travels through the *esophageal hiatus* with the **vagus** nerve at the *T10* level; the vena cava passes through the diaphragm at *T8.*

The three branches of the celiac axis are the **common hepatic, splenic,** and **left gastric.**

Case 28

Anatomy & Embryology

History

A 62-year-old man complains of left-sided facial pain and numbness. The patient says his symptoms started 1 month ago and have been getting worse. He has no significant past medical history, was previously healthy, and takes no medications. Family history is unremarkable.

Physical Exam

The patient has significantly decreased sensation in the lower face involving areas *A, B,* and *C* in the figure. He also has some weakness when trying to clench his teeth, and you note that the left masseter muscle is atrophic compared with the right. The corneal reflex is absent. The rest of the neurological and general physical exam is normal.

Tests

Complete blood count: normal
Electrolytes: normal

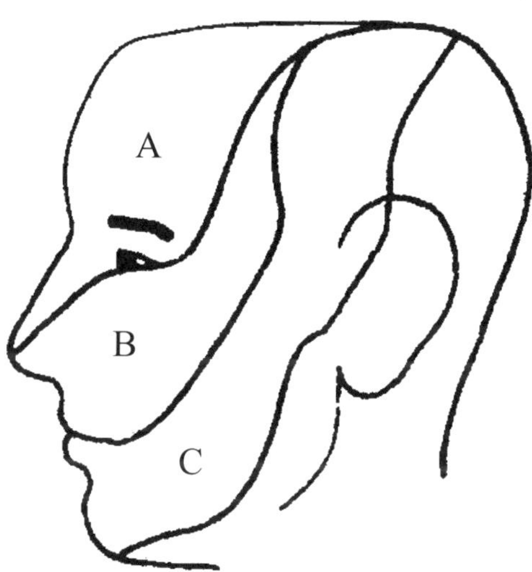

Questions

- What nerves supply sensation to the areas labeled *A, B,* and *C*? From what part of the central nervous system do they arise?
- A lesion to what nerve would cause the muscle weakness and atrophy described in this patient?
- What other structures are innervated by the nerves referred to in the first two questions?

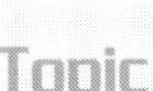

Trigeminal nerve, also known as the fifth cranial nerve (CN V)

Discussion

CN V exits the brainstem from the pons and is the nerve of the first branchial arch. It carries *general sensory afferent* fibers from the skin and mucous membranes of the face, eyes (the **afferent limb of the corneal reflex,** whereas CN VII is the efferent limb) and oral and nasal cavities. It also carries *special visceral efferent* fibers, which supply the **muscles of mastication** (temporalis, masseter, and lateral and medial pterygoid muscles), *tensor tympani, tensor veli palatini, mylohyoid,* and *anterior belly of the digastric muscles.*

CN V has three primary divisions, which have their cell bodies in the *trigeminal (semilunar or gasserian) ganglion* of the middle cranial fossa. The *ophthalmic division (V1)* supplies sensation to area *A* in the figure and enters the orbit via the **superior orbital fissure.** The *maxillary division (V2)* supplies *B* and travels through the **foramen rotundum.** The *mandibular division (V3)* supplies *C* and exits via the **foramen ovale.**

Findings

A lesion of CN V has the potential to cause **loss of facial sensation, loss of the corneal (i.e., blink) reflex,** and **motor weakness** (most apparent clinically when the patient clenches the teeth and the masseter muscle on the affected side is palpated, as in this case).

The cause of this patient's symptoms cannot be ascertained with the given information. A condition called *trigeminal neuralgia* (tic douloureux) can cause episodes of sharp, stabbing pain, typically in older adults in the V3 or V2 region. Its cause is unknown, but motor function remains intact with this condition. Other causes of CN V lesions include stroke, tumor, infection (e.g., herpesvirus), and multiple sclerosis.

More High-Yield Facts

Tongue innervation: CN V supplies general sensation to the *anterior two thirds of the tongue,* but taste to this region is supplied by the facial nerve. The glossopharyngeal nerve (CN IX) supplies general and taste sensation to the *posterior one third of the tongue.* The vagus nerve supplies general and taste sensation to the *epiglottic region of the oral cavity* (just posterior to tongue). All the *intrinsic muscles of the tongue* except the palatoglossus (which is supplied by the vagus nerve) are supplied by the hypoglossal nerve (CN XII).

Four different cranial nerves supply sensation to the outer ear: *trigeminal, facial, glossopharyngeal, and vagus.*

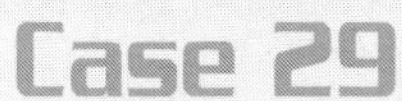

Anatomy & Embryology

History

A 7-year-old girl is brought to your office for a follow-up visit related to newly discovered hypertension. The girl has Turner syndrome, but her medical history is otherwise unremarkable. She takes no medications.

Physical Exam

Cardiovascular exam reveals hypertension in both upper extremities with a normal blood pressure in both lower extremities. The femoral pulses are significantly delayed and diminished compared with the brachial pulses. You hear a systolic murmur over the mid-upper back.

Tests

Complete blood count: normal
Chest x-ray: reveals rib notching bilaterally
MRI of the thoracic aorta: see figure

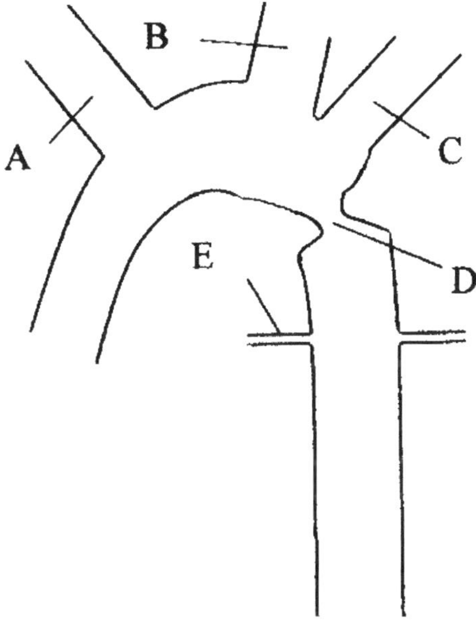

Questions

- Name the three arteries labeled *A, B,* and *C* that arise from the aortic arch.
- What is the abnormality shown at *D* called?
- What important collateral vessels (*E*) hypertrophy in this condition? Describe the collateral pathway these vessels help form.
- To what structures do the six respective embryologic aortic arches give rise?

Topic Thoracic aorta and aortic coarctation

Discussion

The thoracic aortic arch and proximal pulmonary artery arise from the six aortic arches. The three main branches off the aorta are the *brachiocephalic (or innominate) artery* (*A* in the figure), *left common carotid* (*B*) and *left subclavian* (*C*).

Aortic Arch	Structures Formed
First	Maxillary artery
Second	Hyoid and stapedial arteries
Third	**Common and proximal internal carotids**
Fourth	**Proximal right subclavian** and **part of aortic arch**
Fifth	Regresses completely
Sixth	**Proximal pulmonary artery** and **ductus arteriosus**

Findings

One of the aortic anomalies that can occur is *coarctation* (stenosis, *D* in the figure), which usually occurs **just distal to the left subclavian artery origin and ductus arteriosus** (postductal). In some cases, the narrowing occurs in the more proximal aorta (preductal), which usually is detected early in life owing to greater cardiovascular compromise. Postductal narrowing classically results in the development of **upper extremity–only hypertension** with significantly lower blood pressure in the lower extremities and a *delay in the timing of pulses* between the brachial (or radial) and femoral arteries. A systolic murmur also may be present.

Postductal coarctation results in development of collateral circulation between the preductal and postductal aorta to supply the lower extremities with blood. In one pathway, the posterior intercostal branches (*E*) of the postductal aorta anastomose with the anterior intercostal branches of the **internal thoracic arteries** (which arise from the subclavian arteries). Other collaterals form between the *superior epigastric* (one of the two terminal branches of the internal thoracic, along with the musculophrenic) and *inferior epigastric* (branch of external iliac) arteries.

More High-Yield Facts

In long-standing uncorrected coarctation, the hypertrophy of the posterior intercostal arteries can lead to erosion of the lower border of the ribs (where the neurovascular bundle runs). This rib erosion, called **rib notching,** is a sign of coarctation that can be seen on x-ray and primarily affects the third through eighth ribs. The first two posterior intercostal arteries are supplied by the **costocervical trunk** (off the subclavian artery), and thus the first two ribs do not develop notching.

Case 30

Anatomy & Embryology

History

You are asked to evaluate a 2-year-old girl for delayed mental and speech development. The patient was born without difficulty, although the foreign-born mother tells you that she had German measles during the first trimester of the pregnancy. The child's past medical history is significant for some type of congenital heart defect and cataracts that were surgically corrected during infancy. The mother states that the child seems slow to her and has not said her first words, which should occur at 9 to 12 months of age. The mother also thinks her child may be deaf.

Physical Exam

The child is deaf and unable to speak. Motor development also seems delayed, and you note microcephaly.

Tests

Hemoglobin: normal
White blood cell count: normal
Electrolytes: normal

Questions

- Could the history of German measles in the mother be related to the child's problems? What causes German measles?
- What are the major in utero infectious agents represented by the TORCH acronym?
- *True or false:* Children can acquire human immunodeficiency virus (HIV) infection from their mother either in utero or after birth if the mother breast-feeds.
- When is a fetus most susceptible to develop gross birth defects from exposure to a teratogen (what is the name and length of the period)?

Topic In utero infections and the TORCH complex

Discussion

TORCH stands for a group of infectious agents that can be transmitted to a fetus if its mother is infected during pregnancy. Major birth defects can result in some cases.

A fetus is most susceptible to teratogens (agents that cause abnormal fetal development) during the period of **organogenesis,** which occurs **3 to 8 weeks** after conception. Devastating effects still can result from certain agents after this period (e.g., HIV). In utero fetal infections are one group of teratogens; they reach the fetus by *transplacental spread*. Not all infectious agents can cross the placenta (most that can are viruses; bacteria *cannot* cross).

Findings

Intrauterine fetal infections may cause mental retardation, microcephaly, low birth weight, and other problems. The TORCH infections are the classic offenders:

Toxoplasma gondii: a protozoa classically acquired by the mother from exposure to *cats*. May cause cerebral calcifications and mental retardation.
Other: *varicella zoster virus, hepatitis B virus,* and *syphilis.*
Rubella (the cause of German measles): classic triad with first-trimester infection is *cardiovascular defects* (patent ductus arteriosus, ventricular septal defect), *deafness,* and *cataracts.*
Cytomegalovirus: most common; also may cause cerebral calcifications and mental retardation (not associated with cats).
Herpes: classically causes limb hypoplasia and skin scarring, and **HIV,** which can be acquired transplacentally (in utero) or *via breast milk* (women with HIV should not breast-feed).

Prevention & Treatment

Prevention is the best means to treat these disorders: People routinely are immunized against rubella, hepatitis, and varicella-zoster virus; pregnant women can consider avoiding cats during pregnancy; and maternal and infant treatment can lessen transmission rates (e.g., with anti-HIV medications, intravenous hepatitis B immune globulin, cesarean section if the mother has genital herpes lesions).

More High-Yield Facts

Infections in the mother and newborn acquired during gestation may be subclinical and asymptomatic (i.e., birth defects do not always occur), or birth defects (e.g., mental retardation) may not be noticed until later in childhood.

Case 31

Anatomy & Embryology

History

A 2-year-old child presents with a heart murmur. The child had increasing fatigue and was found to have a murmur on physical exam. The patient's mother would like your opinion as to what the cause is and what should be done about it. The child has no significant past medical history and takes no medications.

Physical Exam

Cardiac exam reveals a loud holosystolic murmur best heard adjacent to the lower left sternal border. The remainder of the exam is unremarkable.

Tests

Hemoglobin: normal
White blood cell count: normal
Cardiac ultrasound: reveals a defect/hole in the structure that separates cardiac chambers *C* and *D* in the figure

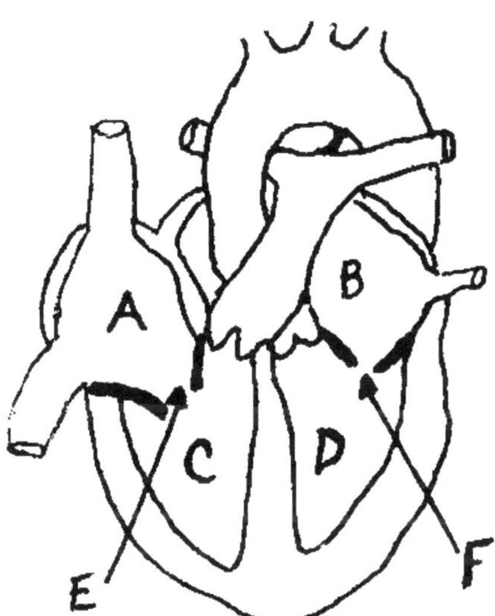

Questions

- Name the cardiac chambers labeled *A* through *D* in the figure.
- Name the heart valves labeled *E* and *F*.
- What is the defect seen on the cardiac ultrasound called?
- Describe the path of a red blood cell (i.e., the structures it normally passes through) as it flows from the vena cava all the way to the aorta in a normal adult.

Topic The heart and septal defects

Discussion

The interatrial septum separates the right and left atria and is formed by the **septum primum** (forms first), the **septum secundum** (forms second), and the *endocardial cushions.* The foramen ovale, which normally closes shortly after birth, is an opening left by the septum secundum to allow oxygenated blood from the placenta to be shunted into the systemic circulation.

The ventricular septum is formed by the **muscular septum,** which forms the lower two thirds of the septum, and the **membranous interventricular septum,** which connects the free edge of the muscular septum with the *endocardial cushions.*

Findings

The most common type of atrial septal defect (ASD) is an **ostium secundum** defect (owing to failure of the septum secundum to close completely), but **ostium primum** defects (owing to failure of septum primum closure) also can occur and are often more severe. Patent foramen ovale is a separate condition that is considered distinct from ASD, although it causes similar pathophysiology. Patients with ASDs are *often asymptomatic until adulthood.* On exam, they classically have a **fixed, split S_2 heart sound** and may have a *diastolic* mumur.

A ventricular septal defect (VSD)—this patient's condition—is usually due to failure of closure in the *membranous portion* of the septum and may involve the endocardial cushions, making it a more complex lesion, although muscular septal defects also can occur. **VSDs are the most common congenital heart defect** and have been associated with *fetal alcohol syndrome, TORCH infections, and Down syndrome.* Patients with VSDs have **holosystolic murmurs** best heard along the lower left sternal border.

Treatment

Treatment for ASDs and VSDs, if needed, is surgical correction. Many VSDs present at birth are small and eventually close on their own.

More High-Yield Facts

In a normal heart, blood flows from returning systemic veins into the *right atrium* (labeled *A* in the figure), then through the *tricuspid valve* (*E*) and into the *right ventricle* (*C*). From the right ventricle, blood flows through the *pulmonic valve* into the *pulmonary artery.* After picking up oxygen from the lungs, blood returns to the *left atrium* (*B*) by way of the *pulmonary veins,* then goes through the *mitral valve* (*F*) into the *left ventricle* (*D*). The left ventricle pumps blood through the aortic valve into the aorta.

Anatomy & Embryology

History

A 12-year-old girl is brought to your office because she has developed multiple "bumps" on her skin. The child's mother died of a rare disorder and the family is not sure what it is called, but the mother also had multiple skin growths, some of which were large and unsightly. The mother ultimately died of a brain tumor. The child is healthy and takes no medications.

Physical Exam

Exam reveals pigmented hamartomas in the iris (Lisch nodules), multiple large light brown café-au-lait macules, and hundreds of soft, subcutaneous nodules and larger pedunculated skin lesions (see figure). The patient has diminished hearing in the right ear on testing.

Tests

Hemoglobin: normal
MRI of the brain: large acoustic neuroma involving the right eighth cranial nerve.

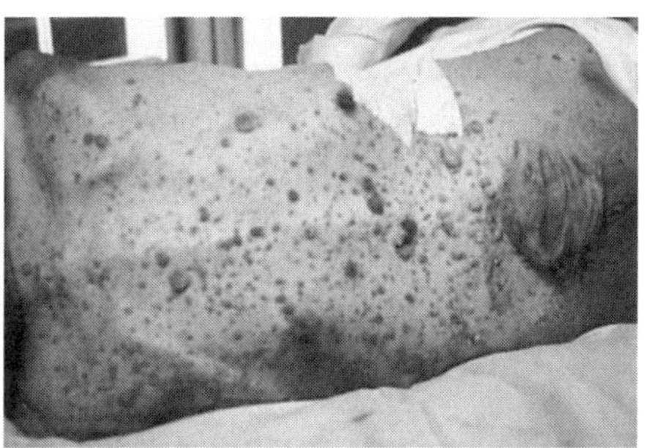

Questions

- What disorder do you suspect this child has?
- Do you think her mother's condition was related? Why or why not (i.e., what is the inheritance pattern of the child's presumed disorder)?
- What chromosome is involved in this disorder?
- What are the skin growths shown in the figure called?

Topic Neurofibromatosis (NF)

Discussion

NF generally is divided into type 1 (NF-1) and type 2 (NF-2). Both disorders are *autosomal dominant* but exhibit *high spontaneous mutation rates* (50%), so that not all affected patients have a family history. NF-1 is much more common than NF-2 and is due to a defect in a gene that codes for **neurofibromin** on **chromosome 17.** This protein is a tumor-suppressor gene that normally down-regulates the function of the p21 *ras* oncoprotein, which has been implicated in multiple tumors. NF-2 also is due to a mutation in a tumor-suppressor gene, but this one is located on **chromosome 22** and is involved in cytoskeleton linkage to membrane proteins.

Findings

Patients are prone to tumor development. The skin tumors, which are seen in most NF-1 patients, are of neural origin (peripheral nerves) and are known as **neurofibromas.** These tumors contain a mixture of *neural tissue, Schwann cells, and fibroblasts*. In addition, patients with either NF-1 or NF-2 may develop **neuromas** (neurilemmomas or schwannomas), which are composed primarily of Schwann cells and, in contrast to neurofibromas, *do not contain neural tissue*. Classically (and commonly), neuromas involve the eighth cranial nerve, which has been termed an *acoustic neuroma* or *acoustic schwannoma*.

The classic skin finding at birth (before neurofibromas have become apparent clinically) in NF-1 patients is the **café-au-lait spot,** a pigmented, brown, flat (i.e., macule) skin "spot"; typically more than five are present. In addition, a *pigmented iris hamartoma,* called a **Lisch nodule,** is usually present in NF-1. Although NF-1 and NF-2 patients can have acoustic neuromas, the nearly pathognomonic finding in NF-2 is **bilateral acoustic neuromas.**

Patients with NF also are at risk for other neoplasms, including pheochromocytomas, meningiomas, and optic nerve gliomas. Neurofibromas have the potential for malignant degeneration.

More High-Yield Facts

The *ras* family of proteins plays an important role in signal transduction leading to cell division. These proteins function by transforming extracellular signals by intracellular effectors, such as phospholipase. Ultimately, the cascade begun by *ras* proteins leads to activation of *cell transcription factors* that are involved in cell division. **Roughly one third of all human cancers** contain one or more mutations in *ras* proteins.

Case 33

Anatomy & Embryology

History

You are asked to give genetic counseling to three different patients with potentially heritable diseases.

Patient 1 has seizures, mild mental retardation, and multiple lesions on his face consistent with adenoma sebaceum. An MRI of his brain reveals abnormal neuronal migration in the brain and multiple nodules in the brain parenchyma that have not grown in years. He has a past history of multiple renal angiomyolipomas and a cardiac rhabdomyoma. The patient's father and grandmother had the same disorder.

Patient 2 has a personal history of cerebellar and retinal hemangioblastomas and bilateral renal cell carcinomas. She also is known to have cysts of the liver and pancreas. The patient's father and grandfather had the same disorder.

Patient 3 has a strong history of nonmelanoma skin cancer on both sides of his family and has had two skin cancers himself. On testing, he is found to have an inherited defect in DNA repair of UV light–induced pyrimidine dimers.

Questions

- What heritable disorders do you think patients 1, 2, and 3 have?
- How are these conditions inherited?
- What is ataxia-telangiectasia? How is it inherited?

Topic Various hereditary forms of neoplasia

Discussion

Although rare, some of the inheritable forms of neoplasia provide important insights into the mechanisms of cancer development and are a favorite topic of board examiners.

Findings

Tuberous sclerosis (patient 1) is an *autosomal dominant* condition characterized by the clinical triad of **adenoma sebaceum, seizures, and mental retardation.** Adenoma sebaceum is a skin disorder with lesions that resemble pimples to some extent and also are called *angiofibromas*. Patients are prone to develop multiple uncommon neoplasms, including **renal angiomyolipomas, cardiac rhabdomyomas,** and **subependymal giant cell astrocytomas.** Affected individuals also commonly develop *central nervous system hamartomas* (called *tubers*), which are the nodules seen on the patient's MRI, and disordered neuronal migration and organization.

Von Hippel–Lindau disease (patient 2) is an *autosomal dominant* condition that leaves patients at risk of developing **retinal and cerebellar hemangioblastomas** (these also can occur in the brainstem and spinal cord); **renal cell carcinoma;** and *cysts in the liver, kidneys, and pancreas*. The abnormal gene has been mapped to *chromosome 3*.

Xeroderma pigmentosum (patient 3) is an *autosomal recessive* condition and affected individuals are at high risk for developing **skin cancer** because of an inherited *defect in repair of UV light–induced pyrimidine dimer formation in DNA*. These dimers, when left unrepaired, can cause transcriptional errors and, in some cases, cancer.

More High-Yield Facts

Ataxia-telangiectasia, an *autosomal recessive* condition, is characterized by **cerebellar ataxia, multiple telangiectasias** in the skin and eyes, and variable immunodeficiency. Patients also have a defective ability to repair damage induced by *ionizing radiation* and are at an increased risk for developing lymphomas.

Fanconi's anemia and **Bloom's syndrome** are two other rare autosomal recessive conditions that lead to an increased risk of various malignancies caused by defective DNA repair mechanisms. In a sense, DNA repair mechanisms can be considered tumor-suppressor genes; generally both gene copies must be damaged to increase significantly the risk of developing malignancies.

Case 34

Anatomy & Embryology

History

A 46-year-old man is brought to the emergency department with sudden onset of severe headaches and altered mental status. The patient complained to his wife that he was having the "worst headache" of his life before he became less responsive and disoriented. The patient's past medical history includes hypertension, and he takes atenolol daily. He is otherwise usually healthy and has no history of head trauma.

Physical Exam

The patient has some neck rigidity and a decreased level of consciousness with disorientation. No focal neurologic deficits are identified, and the physical exam is otherwise unremarkable.

Tests

Complete blood count: normal

Lumbar puncture with cerebrospinal fluid analysis: normal white blood cell count, many red blood cells seen

MRI of the brain: subarachnoid hemorrhage with an aneurysm that appears to be arising from the anterior communicating artery

Diagram of the circle of Willis: see figure

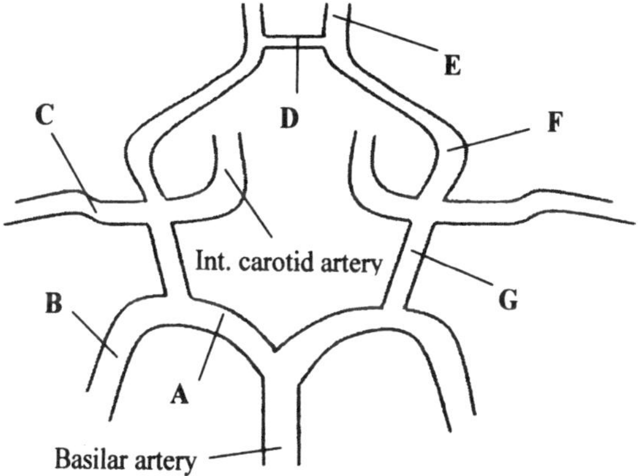

Questions

- From which labeled structure in the diagram does the patient's aneurysm appear to arise?
- What are the other structures labeled *A* through *G* in the figure?
- What two main vessels supply the *anterior* and *posterior* circulation? What do these terms mean?

The circle of Willis

Discussion

The circle of Willis reflects a union of the posterior, anterior, right, and left circulations of the brain and brainstem, which becomes important in times of ischemia. The anterior circulation is supplied by the internal carotid arteries and is the primary blood supply to the cerebral hemispheres. The posterior circulation is supplied by the vertebral arteries and delivers blood to the brainstem and the posterior aspect of the cerebral hemispheres.

The final branches of the internal carotid artery, in order, are the ophthalmic, **posterior communicating artery** (labeled *G* in the figure), and anterior choroidal artery. The internal carotid artery terminates by bifurcating into the *anterior* (*E* and *F* in the figure—yes, this is meant to trick you) and *middle* (*C*) *cerebral arteries*. The anterior cerebral arteries are connected by the **anterior communicating artery** (*D*).

The **basilar artery** is formed by the joining of the **vertebral arteries** after the vertebral arteries give off the *posterior inferior cerebellar arteries*. The basilar gives off several branches (in order, anterior inferior cerebellar arteries, pontine branches, and superior cerebellar arteries) before bifurcating into the two **posterior cerebral arteries** (*A* and *B*—yes, this is meant to trick you). The posterior cerebral arteries each join with a posterior communicating artery branch from the internal carotid artery to complete the circle of Willis.

Findings

Aneurysms, or abnormal dilation of blood vessels, can form in the circle of Willis. These are classically **congenital / berry aneurysms** related to **hypertension** or **adult polycystic kidney disease**. If an aneurysm ruptures, as in this patient, it can cause subarachnoid hemorrhage, stroke, or death. Patients classically complain of the **worst headache of their lives** and have *altered mental status*. Nuchal rigidity (owing to meningeal irritation) and bloody cerebrospinal fluid also are commonly present.

Treatment

Treatment is surgical repair for those who survive.

More High-Yield Facts

The anterior cerebral artery supplies the *medial* portion of the frontal and parietal cortexes; an infarct in this vascular territory commonly causes motor symptoms in the *lower extremities* owing to the location of the neurons supplying them (the homunculus or somatotopic organization of the motor cortex). The middle cerebral artery covers the *lateral* aspect of the frontal and parietal lobes, and infarcts in this territory affect the *upper extremity and face*.

Case 35

Anatomy & Embryology

History

A man presents with double vision. The patient was told he had a small stroke 1 week ago and since that time seems to have double vision that is made worse when he looks to the left. He has a history of hypertension, diabetes, and hypercholesterolemia. He takes enalapril, insulin, and atorvastatin.

Physical Exam

Eye exam reveals symmetric pupils that react normally to accommodation and light. When the patient looks straight ahead, the eyes are normally situated. The patient is unable to look lateral to the midline with his left eye when you tell him to look to the left, although the right eye turns normally toward the midline (see figure). All other extraocular muscles and movements are intact. The rest of the exam is normal.

Tests

Complete blood count: normal
Erythrocyte sedimentation rate: normal

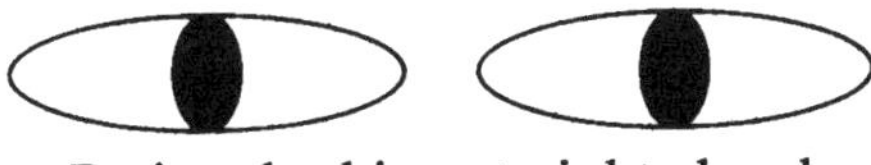

Patient looking straight ahead

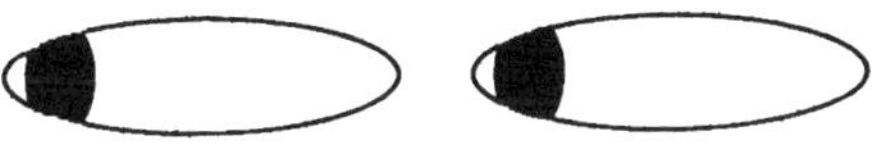

Patient asked to look to the right

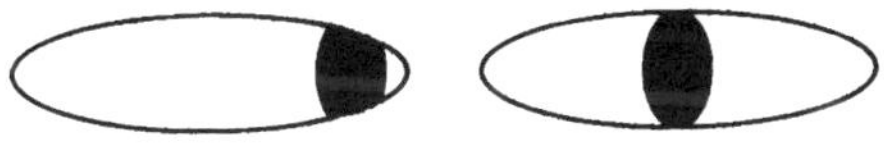

Patient asked to look to the left

Questions:

- A lesion to what cranial nerve is the likely cause of this patient's findings?
- What are the three cranial nerves involved in moving the eye? What muscles do these nerves innervate?
- What cranial nerves regulate pupil size? What are the clinical findings of Horner's syndrome, and what causes this syndrome?
- What cranial nerves make up the corneal reflex? Which is afferent, and which is efferent?

Topic Innervation of the eye

Discussion

The patient in this case has a left cranial nerve (CN) VI or abducent palsy. CN II through VII innervate ocular structures. CN II (optic nerve) carries visual information from the retina in special somatic afferent fibers. CN III (oculomotor), IV (trochlear), and VI (abducent) supply motor function to the extraocular muscles. CN III also supplies the levator palpebrae muscle of the eyelid and carries preganglionic parasympathetic fibers from the **Edinger-Westphal** nucleus to the *ciliary ganglion.* Postganglionic parasympathetic fibers supply the *constrictor muscles of the iris* (i.e., sphincter pupillae muscles) and *ciliary muscles*—parasympathetic stimulation causes **pupillary constriction** and **accommodation.**

Sympathetic fibers course from T1–T2 up to synapse in the **superior cervical ganglion,** then postganglionic fibers travel along the carotid and ophthalmic arteries to supply the **tarsal muscles of Mueller** in the eyelids and the **dilator pupillae muscles** of the iris (sympathetic stimulation causes **elevation of the lid** and **pupillary dilation**).

Findings

CN III supplies the *medial, superior, and inferior rectus muscles* and the *inferior oblique muscle.* CN IV supplies the *superior oblique muscle,* whereas CN VI supplies the *lateral rectus muscle* (mnemonic: the chemical formula LR_6SO_4). A CN III lesion causes the eye to **look "down and out"** (laterally and slightly inferiorly) **at rest,** owing to unopposed tone in the superior oblique and lateral rectus muscles. In the affected eye, patients **can look only laterally.** Patients also develop mild ptosis (levator palpebrae paralysis), and damage to parasympathetic fibers causes a fixed, dilated (mydriasis) pupil and loss of accommodation.

CN IV lesions cause **weakness of downward gaze** (worse when the gaze is medial on the affected side) and double vision that worsens when trying to look down (**vertical diplopia**). CN VI lesions result in **paralysis of lateral gaze** in the affected eye and double vision that worsens when looking toward the side of the lesion (**horizontal diplopia**). CN V (afferent or sensory limb) and VII (efferent or motor limb) make up the corneal reflex.

More High-Yield Facts

Horner's syndrome is a lesion of the ascending sympathetic neurons to the eye and face, classically by apical lung cancer (i.e., **Pancoast tumor**). This syndrome can result in ipsilateral **miosis** (owing to unopposed parasympathetic tone on the iris), **ptosis** (owing to paralysis of tarsal lid muscles of Mueller), and **hemianhidrosis** (absent sweating on affected side of face, which is regulated by sympathetic fibers).

Case 36

Anatomy & Embryology

History

A 56-year-old woman presents to the emergency department with severe abdominal pain and nausea. The patient is normally healthy and says her pain began several hours ago and continues to get worse. The pain is generalized and accompanied by nausea. The patient denies weight loss but thinks she may have a mild fever. Past medical history is essentially unremarkable, and the patient denies prior episodes of pain.

Physical Exam

Vital signs are normal other than a low-grade fever. The abdomen is soft but tender diffusely. No peritoneal signs are present.

Tests

Complete blood count: mild leukocytosis, otherwise normal
Abdominal CT scan: axial images with intravenous and oral contrast (see figures)

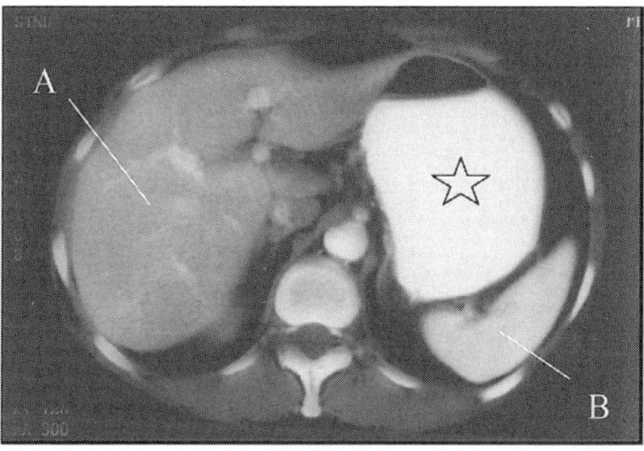

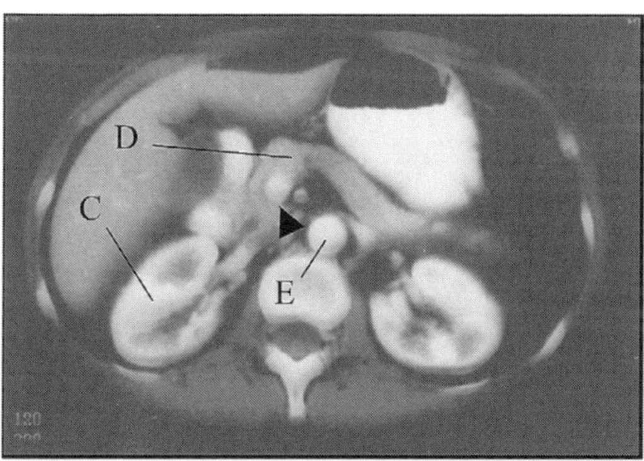

Question

- What are the major structures and organs labeled *A* through *E* in the figures?

CT abdominal anatomy

Discussion

Cross-sectional imaging, including CT, MRI, and ultrasound, is used increasingly to screen for and analyze disease. Imaging also helps to improve your understanding of anatomy and makes for great board questions to ensure that you understand the relationship of major anatomic structures that are important in clinical medicine.

On a CT scan, oral and intravenous contrast agents can be given, which both show up as *white* on the image. The large structure labeled with an asterisk between the liver (the liver is labeled *A* in the first figure) and the spleen (*B*) is the stomach, which is *filled with contrast material.* The aorta (*E*) also is filled with contrast material and appears white. The kidneys (*C*) can be seen in the second image, as can the pancreas (*D*).

In standard cross-sectional *axial* images, **the patient's right is on the left side of the image,** and the *anterior aspect of the patient is at the top of the image.* The spine can be seen just below the aorta in the images because it lies more posterior than the aorta. It is as if the patient is lying on his or her back and we are looking up toward the head while standing at the patient's feet.

Other things to remember on a CT scan are that *air shows up as black,* and *bone and calcium show up as white* (just like on a plain x-ray). Fluid is dark gray whereas most soft tissues (e.g., muscles, liver) are light gray.

More High-Yield Facts

The left renal vein is longer than the right and must pass anterior to the aorta and *between the aorta and the origin of the superior mesenteric artery* to reach the inferior vena cava.

The superior mesenteric vein (*arrowhead* in second figure) and superior mesenteric artery (in the CT scan, the smaller vessel just to the right [or to the patient's left] of the superior mesenteric vein) can be identified in part because of their relationship to the pancreas. The **uncinate process** of the pancreas hooks around just posterior to the origin of the superior mesenteric vessels, as shown in the CT scan.

Case 37

Anatomy & Embryology

History

A mother brings her 18-month-old son into your office for easy bruising. The mother states that her son has developed multiple severe bruises from seemingly minor trauma ever since he began walking several months ago. In addition, last week the mother noticed that her son bled heavily after sustaining a minor cut on his arm. The child is otherwise healthy and takes no medications. The mother mentions that her brother, from whom she is estranged and has not seen since she was a child, had a severe bleeding and bruising tendency that required repeated medical treatment.

Physical Exam

The child is alert and playful but has multiple large, deep bruises in several areas of his body. The remainder of the exam is unremarkable, and the child is not tender in any of the bruised areas.

Tests

Hemoglobin: normal
Platelet count: normal
Prothrombin time (PT): normal
Partial thromboplastin time (PTT): prolonged
Bleeding time: normal
Factor levels: all normal except factor VIII, which is low
Antinuclear antibody titer: normal

Questions:

- What condition does this child have? How is it inherited?
- How do the PT and PTT relate to the intrinsic and extrinsic coagulation pathways? What does the bleeding time measure?
- What is the mechanism of action of heparin and warfarin? Which affects the PT, and which affects the PTT?

Hemophilia and the coagulation cascade

Discussion

The coagulation cascade is complex and painful to memorize (but often tested). In the intrinsic pathway, which is initiated by trauma to the blood vessel or exposure of blood to collagen (from a traumatized blood vessel), successive activation of factors XII, XI, IX, VII, X, and V results in activation of prothrombin (or factor II) into **thrombin.**

In the extrinsic pathway, tissue trauma causes release of tissue *thromboplastin,* which interacts with factor VII to activate factor X, which can activate prothrombin into thrombin with the help of factor V. Calcium is required in both pathways, and the end result of each pathway, thrombin, can convert fibrinogen into **fibrin,** which forms a meshlike tangle of threads that are the early basis of clot formation.

Findings

Hemophilia A, or classic hemophilia, is an inherited **X-linked recessive** disorder and affects males almost exclusively. Women are silent carriers and pass the condition on to their sons (but not their daughters); men cannot transmit the disorder to their sons, but will invariably pass on the trait to their daughters. Hemophilia A results in low levels of **factor VIII** and a strong bruising and bleeding tendency. **Hemophilia B,** which is much less common, is also *X-linked recessive* but results in low levels of **factor IX** and similar clinical findings.

The *PT* is used to measure the extrinsic pathway and to monitor the effect of **heparin.** Heparin combines with **antithrombin III** and increases its effectiveness > 100-fold, resulting in the removal of thrombin and inhibition of clot formation. The *PTT* is used to measure the intrinsic pathway and monitor the effects of **warfarin.** Warfarin is a *vitamin K antagonist;* it prevents the formation of the vitamin K–dependent factors **II (prothrombin), VII, IX, and X.**

More High-Yield Facts

The *bleeding time* is a measure of platelet function and is prolonged by **aspirin** and other antiplatelet agents. It rarely is used clinically; however, it is prolonged in **von Willebrand disease** (along with the PTT).

In an emergency, heparin can be reversed by giving **protamine sulfate,** whereas warfarin can be reversed by giving vitamin K or by giving fresh frozen plasma. Warfarin is *teratogenic* and given orally; heparin is given parenterally. *Low-molecular weight heparins (e.g., enoxaparin) do not affect the PTT.*

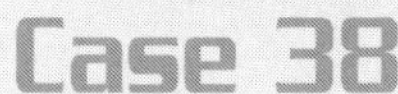

Anatomy & Embryology

History

A 62-year-old man presents with vertigo and hearing loss. The patient states that he has had gradual onset of hearing loss in his right ear and a sensation that the room is spinning around him over the last month or so. He is otherwise healthy and takes no medications.

Physical Exam

When you whisper next to the patient's ears, you notice that the patient definitely can hear better in his left ear compared with his right. You place a vibrating tuning fork on the vertex of the patient's skull. The patient says he hears the sound of the tuning fork louder in his left ear.

You then place a vibrating tuning fork over both mastoid processes until the sound can no longer be heard. When the sound can no longer be heard, you move the tuning fork and hold it in front of the respective ear. On the right, the patient hears the vibration next to his ear after he can no longer hear the tuning fork while it is held over the mastoid, but only briefly. On the left, the patient hears the tuning fork next to his ear (after he can no longer hear it while it is over the mastoid) for a much longer time compared with the right. The patient also has an unsteady gait.

Tests

Complete blood count: normal
Erythrocyte sedimentation rate: normal

Questions:

- What cranial nerve is involved in hearing? A lesion to which cranial nerve can cause vertigo?
- Does this patient have sensorineural hearing loss or conduction deafness?
- What are the Weber and Rinne tests, and how are they performed and interpreted?
- What is presbycusis? Does it relate to conduction or sensorineural hearing loss?

Topic Cranial nerve (CN) VIII

Discussion

CN VIII arises from the pons, exits the brainstem at the *cerebellopontine angle,* and enters the internal auditory canal along with the facial nerve. It consists of two major divisions: the **cochlear** and **vestibular.** The cochlear nerve is involved in hearing and innervates the **hair cells in the organ of Corti** with special somatic afferent fibers. The vestibular nerve is involved in balance and supplies the **hair cells in the vestibular labyrinth** with special somatic afferent fibers.

Lesions of CN VIII can cause sensorineural *hearing loss* or **tinnitus** (ringing in the ears) or both if the cochlear division is affected or **vertigo** (a sensation of an irregular or whirling motion while at rest), dysequilibrium, and **nystagmus** if the vestibular division is involved. Classic lesions affecting CN VIII include **presbycusis,** a normal part of aging that affects the cochlear division and results in high-frequency range hearing loss, and *acoustic neuromas.*

Findings

The Weber and Rinne tests are important physical exam maneuvers to help determine the type and cause of hearing loss. There are two primary types of hearing loss: **sensorineural,** resulting from CN VIII damage or irritation, and **conductive,** resulting from blockage to the passage of sound waves into the inner ear (e.g., wax in the ears, otitis media, and otosclerosis). In the **Weber test,** a vibrating tuning fork is placed on the forehead or vertex of the skull. The sound of the tuning fork normally is heard equally in both ears. The sound is heard better, however, on the affected side with conductive hearing (loss) and on the unaffected side with sensorineural hearing loss.

In the **Rinne test,** a vibrating tuning fork is placed over the mastoid (bone conduction [BC]) until the patient can no longer hear its sound, then the tuning fork is held next to the ear (air conduction [AC]) on the same side to determine if the patient can hear the sound of the tuning fork. Normally, AC > BC, and this relationship is maintained in sensorineural hearing loss (although the patient has impaired AC and BC overall). In conductive hearing loss, however, BC > AC, and patients cannot hear the tuning fork when it is moved next to their ear.

The patient in this case has right-sided sensorineural hearing loss.

More High-Yield Facts

Aminoglycosides are the classic antibiotic cause of drug-induced deafness. Quinine, **aspirin,** in utero rubella infection, meningitis, and prolonged exposure to loud noises are other causes of sensorineural hearing loss.

Case 39

Anatomy & Embryology

History

An embryologist is studying fetal growth and development of the central nervous system. The embryologist experimentally alters development in several fetuses to determine which structures depend on which embryologic remnants.

At various stages of development, the researcher destroys major portions of the developing nervous system, including the metencephalon, telencephalon, myelencephalon, diencephalon and mesencephalon.

Questions

- Match the central nervous system structures (1–10) to their regions of the developing system (A–E).

1. Cerebral cortex
2. Basal ganglia
3. Cerebellum
4. Thalamus
5. Midbrain
6. Pons
7. Hypothalamus
8. Medulla
9. Cerebral aqueduct
10. Optic chiasm

A. Telencephalon
B. Metencephalon
C. Myelencephalon
D. Diencephalon
E. Mesencephalon

- What main structure gives rise to the telencephalon and the diencephalon?
- What main structure gives rise to the metencephalon and myelencephalon?

Matching answers:
1A, 2A and D, 3B, 4D, 5E, 6B, 7D, 8C, 9E, 10D

Discussion

The three primary brain vesicles that first form in the rostral neural tube begin the differentiation of the central nervous system. These are the **prosencephalon** (forebrain), **mesencephalon** (midbrain), and **rhombencephalon** (hindbrain).

The prosencephalon gives rise to the **telencephalon** and the **diencephalon.** The telencephalon gives rise to the *cerebral cortex, hippocampal formation, amygdala, basal ganglia, olfactory nerves (cranial nerve [CN] I), caudate nucleus, putamen,* and the *lateral ventricles.* The diencephalon gives rise to the *thalamus, hypothalamus, third ventricle, pituitary gland, globus pallidus* (the question that asks about the origin of the basal ganglia is a trick question), and *optic nerve* (CN II), chiasm, and retina.

The **mesencephalon** gives rise to the *midbrain, cerebral aqueduct, and primary nuclei of CN III and IV.* The rhombencephalon gives rise to the **metencephalon** and **myelencephalon.** The metencephalon gives rise to the *pons; cerebellum;* and main nuclei of *CN V, VI, VII, and VIII.* The myelencephalon gives rise to the *medulla oblongata* and the major nuclei of *CN IX, X, XI, and XIII.*

The basal ganglia are the subcortical nuclei located within the cerebral hemispheres and have some confusing terms associated with them:
Striatum (i.e., neostriatum): caudate nucleus and putamen, which have a similar origin from the telencephalon.
Lentiform nucleus: the putamen and globus pallidus (together resemble a lens).
Corpus striatum: the lentiform nucleus (i.e., putamen and globus pallidus) and the caudate nucleus.

The *amygdala, claustrum, substantia nigra, and subthalamic nucleus* also are variably considered basal ganglia, but different texts classify these structures differently. Clinically, many people are referring only to the caudate, globus pallidus, and putamen when they use the term *basal ganglia.*

More High-Yield Facts

Hemiballismus is a curious phenomenon that results from a lesion in the **subthalamic nucleus.** The term describes violent flinging movements of an extremity.

Case 40

Anatomy & Embryology

History

A 31-year-old woman complains of numbness and weakness in her right leg after an injury. The patient had a combination of penetrating and blunt trauma to the lateral aspect of her right leg near the level of the knee with an associated fracture of the neck of the fibula. Her past medical history is unremarkable, and she takes no medications.

Physical Exam

The patient has decreased sensation in her anterolateral leg down into her dorsal foot (in the distribution labeled *A* in the figure). She also has footdrop on the right, with inability to dorsiflex or evert her right foot.

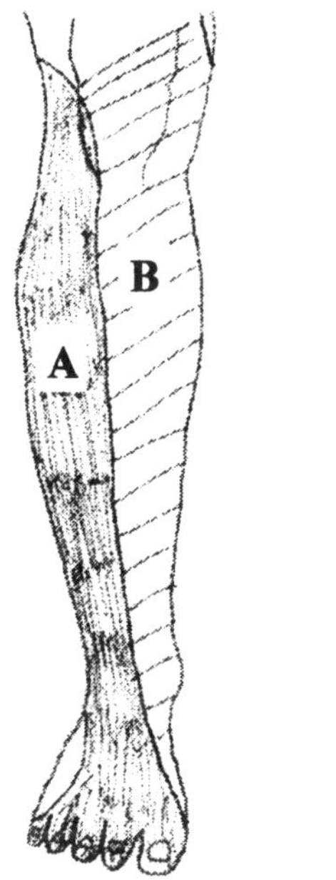

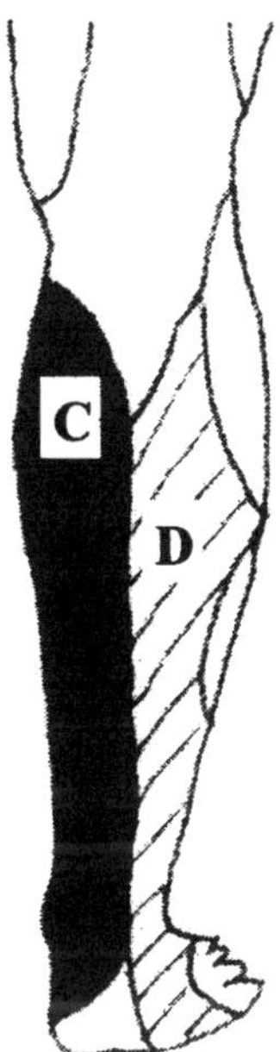

Questions

- Name the nerves that supply cutaneous innervation to the leg in the distributions labeled *A* through *D* in the figure.
- Damage to what major nerve is suggested by the patient's physical exam findings?
- What nerve innervates the anterior and lateral muscles of the leg? What nerve innervates the posterior muscles of the leg?

Innervation of the leg

Discussion

The **sciatic nerve,** which is the *largest nerve in the body* and receives information from cord roots L4 through S3, bifurcates into the **common peroneal** and **tibial** nerves posterior to the knee at the apex of the popliteal fossa. The common peroneal nerve bifurcates into the superficial and deep peroneal nerves.

The tibial nerve supplies the *posterior muscles of the leg,* which are the *primary leg and foot flexors.* These muscles include the gastrocnemius, soleus, plantaris, popliteus, flexor hallicus longus, flexor digitorum longus and tibialis posterior. The tibial nerve also innervates all the muscles of the foot except the *extensor digitorum brevis and extensor hallucis brevis,* which are innervated by the deep peroneal branch of the peroneal nerve.

The peroneal nerve innervates the *anterior and lateral muscles of the leg,* which are the *primary leg extensors and foot dorsiflexors and evertors.* The muscles include the tibialis anterior, extensor hallucis longus, extensor digitorum longus, and peroneus tertius, all supplied by the **deep peroneal** branch. The **superficial peroneal** branch supplies the *peroneus longus* and *peroneus brevis,* which are the primary everters of the foot.

Cutaneous sensation to the medial aspect of the leg (distributions *B* and *C* in the figure) is primarily through the **saphenous nerve,** which is a branch of the femoral nerve. The anterolateral aspect of the leg (distribution *A*) is supplied by the peroneal nerve through the lateral sural cutaneous branch superiorly and by the superficial peroneal nerve inferiorly. The posterolateral aspect of the leg (distribution *D*) is supplied by the tibial nerve through the medial sural cutaneous and sural nerve branches.

More High-Yield Facts

A lesion to the common peroneal trunk, which the patient in this case has, results in **footdrop** and a foot held in an inverted position, with **lack of ability to dorsiflex or evert the foot.** In addition, there is loss of sensation on the dorsum of the foot and lateral aspect of the leg.

A tibial nerve lesion, which is rare clinically, results in **loss of plantar flexion of the foot** and impaired foot inversion. Patients develop a characteristic **clawing of the toes** and may have loss of sensation of the posterolateral aspect of the leg if the cutaneous branches are involved.

Case 41

Anatomy & Embryology

History

A newborn infant develops gagging and cyanosis after every feeding attempt. The mother states that her infant seems hungry, but coughs and gags during attempted feedings. The pregnancy and delivery went smoothly. There are no health problems that run in the family.

Physical Exam

The infant has excessive accumulation of saliva in his mouth. No gross abnormalities are otherwise detected. Attempts to pass a catheter into the stomach are unsuccessful—the catheter seems to get hung up within the upper esophagus with each attempt. X-rays show a large amount of air in the stomach.

Surgery

The infant is taken to surgery and an abnormal connection is noted between the trachea and esophagus. What the surgeon sees is represented in one of the figures.

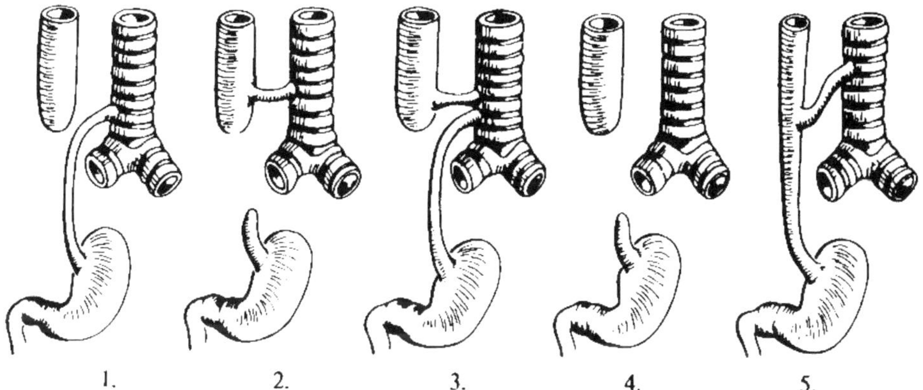

Questions:

- What is the name of this infant's condition?
- The infant has the most common form of this condition—which numbered figure shows the most common type?
- Embryologically, how does this condition develop?

Topic Tracheoesophageal fistula (TEF)

Discussion

The respiratory system begins as an outgrowth from the ventral wall of the primitive **foregut.** Eventually the connection between the trachea and esophagus (a foregut derivative) closes by fusion of the **esophagotracheal ridges.** Because of its foregut origin, the lining epithelium of the respiratory tract is derived from *endoderm.*

If the tracheoesophageal septum improperly divides the foregut, a TEF can occur. A **fistula** is any abnormal connection between two hollow organs or a hollow organ and the skin surface. In most cases, a TEF coexists with *esophageal atresia,* which is depicted in figure 1; this is what the patient in the case has and is the most common variant (85–90% of cases).

Findings

Other tracheoesophageal malformations are depicted in the numbered figures; the second most common variant is esophageal atresia without a TEF (figure 4). Classically, newborns present with **choking, coughing, and cyanosis during attempts at feeding.** Secretions and ingested fluid fill up the blind-ending esophagus and spill over into the back of the throat, causing aspiration into the trachea. **Excessive saliva accumulation** also is noted when the infant is not feeding.

Another classic clinical finding is *inability to pass a catheter through the mouth and esophagus into the stomach.* Distention of the stomach also can occur during crying because of the connection of the airway with the esophagus.

Treatment

Treatment is surgical correction.

More High-Yield Facts

TEF may be part of the **VACTERL** spectrum of disorders. VACTERL is an acronym for the following anomalies that commonly coexist: **v**ertebral anomalies, **a**norectal malformations (e.g., rectal atresia, imperforate anus), **c**ardiac defects, **t**racheoesophageal fistula/**e**sophageal atresia, **r**enal and **l**imb anomalies.

Esophageal atresia is a cause of **polyhydramnios** (excessive accumulation of amniotic fluid) during pregnancy because the fetus is unable to swallow amniotic fluid.

The foregut also gives rise to the stomach, proximal duodenum, liver, gallbladder, bile ducts, and pancreas.

Case 42

Anatomy & Embryology

History

A 22-year-old man suffers severe head trauma during a motor vehicle accident. The patient's past medical history is unknown.

Physical Exam

The patient has an obvious right temporal bone fracture (see figure), decreased level of consciousness, and cannot hear in his right ear.

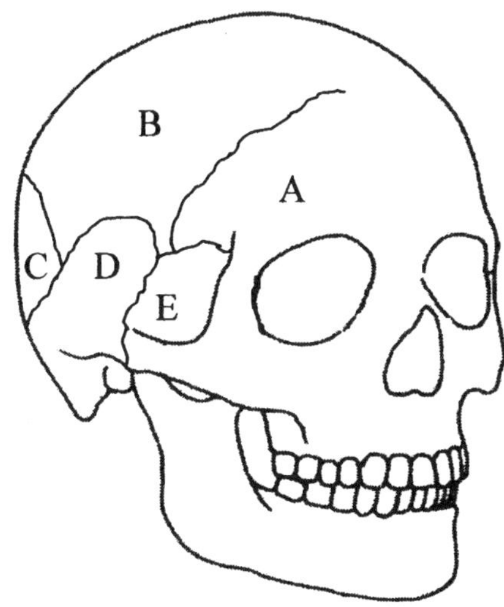

Questions

- In the figure, name the labeled major bones of the skull.
- What artery is classically damaged with a temporal bone fracture and can result in an epidural hematoma/hemorrhage? What foramen does this artery pass through?
- Match the lettered skull foramina with the numbered structures on the left:

1. Abducens nerve (CN VI)
2. Vagus nerve (CN X)
3. Internal carotid artery
4. Olfactory nerve (CN I)
5. Vertebral arteries
6. Glossopharyngeal nerve (CN IX)
7. Oculomotor nerve (CN III)

A. Foramen lacerum
B. Cribriform plate
C. Superior orbital fissure
D. Jugular foramen
E. Foramen magnum
F. Internal acoustic meatus

Matching answers:
1C, 2D, 3A, 4B, 5E, 6D, 7C

Skull bones and foramina

Discussion

The major bones of the skull include the *frontal* (labeled *A* in the figure), *parietal (B), sphenoid (E), temporal (D) and occipital (C)*. The skull foramina course through the sphenoid, temporal, and occipital bones, with the exception of the **cribriform plate** (part of the **ethmoid** bone), through which the fibers of the *olfactory nerve* pass.

The skull often is divided into two parts: the **calvaria,** also called the *dome or vault of the skull,* and the **skull base.** The bulk of the calvaria is formed by the frontal and parietal bones. The skull base includes portions of the frontal, ethmoid, temporal, sphenoid, and occipital bones and is divided into the anterior, middle, and posterior fossae.

The *anterior cranial fossa* houses the **frontal lobes** and extends from the frontal bone anteriorly to the lesser wing of the sphenoid bone posteriorly. From here, the *middle cranial fossa,* which houses the **temporal lobes,** extends back to the superior aspects of the petrous portion of the temporal bone. The *posterior cranial fossa* covers the remainder of the base of the skull and houses the **pons, medulla,** and **cerebellum.**

Other Skull Foramina and Their Contents

FORAMEN (PART OF SKULL)	CONTENTS
Optic canal (S)	Cranial nerve (CN) II, ophthalmic artery, retinal vein
Sup. orbital fissure (S)	CN III, IV, V_1, VI; ophthalmic vein
Foramen rotundum (S)	CN V_2
Foramen ovale (S)	CN V_3
Foramen lacerum (S/T)	Internal carotid artery
Int. acoustic meatus (T)	CN VII, VIII
Jugular foramen (T/O)	CN IX, X, XI; Jugular vein
Foramen magnum (O)	Medulla, vertebral arteries, spinal roots of CN XI
Hypoglossal canal (O)	CN XII

S = sphenoid bone, T = temporal bone, O = occipital bone; two letters means foramen is between the two bones.

More High-Yield Facts

A fracture of the temporal bone can be associated with an **epidural hematoma/ hemorrhage.** Of epidural hematomas, 80–90% are associated with a temporal bone fracture, in large part owing to injury of the **middle meningeal artery.** This artery is a branch of the maxillary artery and courses through the **foramen spinosum** (part of the sphenoid bone), then travels on the undersurface of the temporal bone to supply the dura mater.

Case 43

Anatomy & Embryology

History

A 27-year-old man complains of arm weakness after a motorcycle accident. The patient tells you he was thrown from his motorcycle at a fairly high speed and landed on his left shoulder, with his head bent to the right during his landing. His weakness started right after the accident, which was a few months ago. He did not see a physician before because he thought his symptoms would go away.

Physical Exam

When the patient is standing in a relaxed posture, his left arm hangs limply by his side in medial rotation with the fingers pointing backward and the forearm pronated, as shown in the figure. The patient is unable to initiate abduction of his left shoulder, has weakness of shoulder and arm flexion, and has weakness of forearm supination. The patient also has lost sensation over the lateral arm.

Tests

Complete blood count: normal

Questions

- What condition does the patient have? Injury to what part of the brachial plexus causes this patient's condition?
- Why does this patient have trouble with shoulder abduction? Shoulder flexion? Arm flexion? Supination? Why does he have loss of sensation over the lateral arm?
- A lesion to what nerve causes winging of the scapula? What muscle is affected?

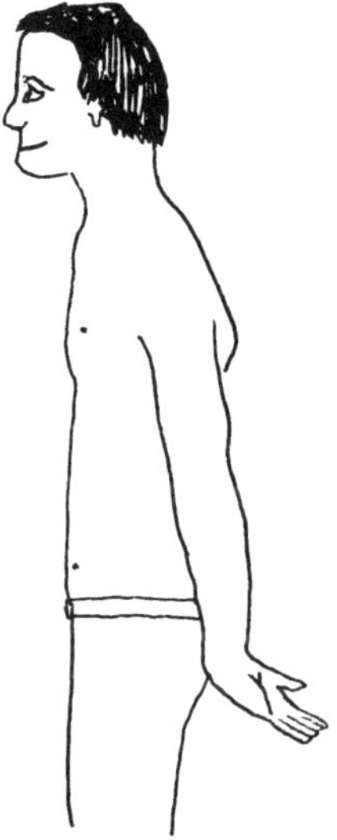

Brachial plexus

Discussion

The brachial plexus is formed by the ventral rami (roots) of *C5 through T1,* which coalesce to form the superior, middle, and inferior trunks. These trunks divide into three anterior and three posterior divisions that form the three cords of the brachial plexus: *lateral, posterior and medial.* The cords are so named because of their relationship to the axillary artery. The lateral cord gives rise to the musculocutaneous nerve and contributes to the formation of the median nerve along with the medial cord, which also gives rise to the ulnar nerve. The posterior cord gives rise to the radial nerve.

Erb-Duchenne palsy, which this patient has, results from a lesion in the *upper* brachial plexus, generally from violent injuries that cause a blow to or fall on a shoulder, with displacement of the head from the shoulder. Birth injuries and *falls from a motorcycle or horse* are classic. The end result is damage to the C5 and C6 nerve roots of the brachial plexus.

Findings

Affected patients develop paralysis of muscles supplied by the *musculocutaneous and axillary nerves.* This includes the supraspinatus and deltoid muscles; thus patients cannot abduct the shoulder. The biceps brachii (arm flexor and forearm supinator), brachialis (arm flexor), and coracobrachialis (shoulder flexor) also are paralyzed or weak, and **the limb hangs limply at the side with the forearm pronated.** The arm also is **medially rotated** at rest because of weakness or paralysis of the primary lateral shoulder rotators, the infraspinatus and teres minor. Finally, there is decreased sensation over much of the lateral aspect of the limb, which is supplied in part by the musculocutaneous (forearm) and axillary (upper arm) nerves.

More High-Yield Facts

The **long thoracic nerve,** supplied by nerve roots from C5–C7, supplies the **serratus anterior** muscle. A lesion to this nerve produces **winging of the scapula,** which describes posterior protrusion of the medial and inferior borders of the scapula. Affected patients also have difficulty raising the arm above the head.

Klumpke's paralysis is due to lesions of the *lower* brachial plexus, involving the *T1* root, typically secondary to *traumatic birth injury* or excessive or violent arm abduction or both. The first thoracic nerve travels within the median and ulnar nerves to supply all the *small muscles of the hand,* and affected patients have a **clawed appearance of the hands.** There is also variable loss of sensation along the medial arm.

Case 44

Anatomy & Embryology

History

A 32-year-old man comes to the office for a routine checkup. The patient has no complaints; no significant past medical history, other than mild dyslexia; and takes no regular medications. He mentions that he and his wife have been trying to conceive a child for the past 4 years unsuccessfully. The patient does not smoke or drink alcohol.

Physical Exam

The patient is quite tall and thin with long legs and a youthful appearance. He has little facial and axillary hair. He has female-like enlargement of the breasts bilaterally, but the chest exam is otherwise unremarkable. Genitalia exam reveals unusually small and firm testicles with a normal-appearing penis. No other abnormalities are identified, although you suspect the patient has mildly decreased intelligence.

Tests

Hemoglobin: normal
White blood cell count: normal
Antinuclear antibody: negative
Testosterone level: low
Follicule-stimulating hormone (FSH): elevated
Buccal smear: occasional cells that contain Barr bodies

Questions:

- What chromosomal disorder does this patient likely have?
- What is the relationship between this disorder and fertility?
- Why is the patient's FSH level elevated?

Topic Klinefelter's syndrome (KS)

Discussion

KS generally describes males with a **47, XXY karyotype,** although some may have a **mosaic-type pattern** or more than two X chromosomes. The cause is most commonly **paternal meiotic nondisjunction,** or uneven chromosome distribution between dividing gametes, leading to *aneuploidy* (an abnormal number of chromosomes). Patients are *psychologically and physically male* but often have multiple mild abnormalities. KS proves that sex in humans is *determined by the presence (males) or absence (females) of a Y chromosome.*

Findings

KS patients are generally **tall** and have **decreased body hair** (especially **facial** and **axillary** hair). The **testes** are **small (< 2 cm) and firm;** contain *hyalinized, nonfunctional testicular tubules;* and *fail to produce sperm* (i.e., **azoospermia**), leading to **infertility. Gynecomastia** (female-like breast development) also is common. The average IQ is mildly decreased in KS patients, but mental retardation is **uncommon.**

The classic presentation is for **delayed sexual development,** decreased sexual function, or **infertility,** although patients may present for unrelated complaints. Lab testing generally reveals **Barr bodies** (usually only present in women and caused by the second X chromosome) and **absence of sperm** in a semen sample. Infertility cannot be corrected in KS because the seminiferous tubules are unable to produce sperm.

KS patients have **decreased testosterone levels** and **elevated gonadotropin** (i.e., FSH and luteinizing hormone [LH]) **levels.** Normally, testosterone (made by *Leydig* cells) and **inhibin** (made by *Sertoli* cells) cause feedback inhibition of LH and FSH, respectively. This inhibition (and testosterone production) is lost in KS, so gonadotropin levels rise in an attempt to stimulate the nonfunctional testes, similar to when the ovaries stop making eggs at menopause in women.

More High-Yield Facts

The **androgen insensitivity syndrome** (i.e., testicular feminization) describes individuals with a **46, XY genotype,** who are *phenotypically and psychologically female.* This disorder is due to an *X-linked recessive* mutation in the *androgen receptor* gene, making it unresponsive to 5α–dihydrotestosterone, resulting in failure of differentiation of external male genitalia. Although patients have an external female appearance, they fail to develop internal genital structures (i.e., no uterus) and have testicular tissue. Patients often present when they *fail to menstruate* and are *infertile.*

Case 45

Anatomy & Embryology

History

A 31-year-old woman complains of right foot pain after an injury. The patient says that another player stepped on her right foot during a soccer game, and it has been hurting ever since. Her past medical history is unremarkable.

Physical Exam

The patient has full range of motion, normal motor function, and no loss of sensation in either lower extremity. She has tenderness over the dorsal aspect of her foot.

Tests

Complete blood count: normal
Schematic of the bones of the feet: see figure

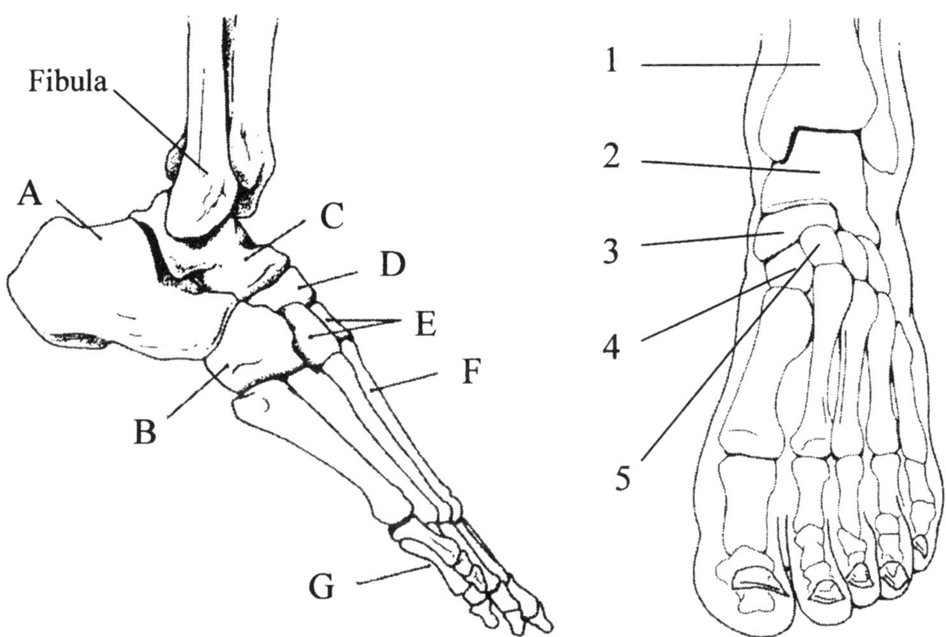

Questions

- Name the structures labeled *A* through *G* and *1* through *5* in the figure.
- What forms the lateral and medial malleolus?
- The pulse of which artery can be felt posterior to the medial malleolus?
- Which artery's pulse can be palpated at the medial aspect of the dorsum of the foot? This artery is a branch of which major leg artery?

Topic Bones of the foot and ankle

Discussion

The ankle joint is formed by the articulation of the inferior ends of the tibia and fibula with the **talus** (labeled *C* and *2* in the figure). The talus articulates with the **calcaneus** (*A*), or heel bone, and **navicular** bones (*D* and *3*). The calcaneus also articulates with the **cuboid** (*B*) and navicular bones.

The lateral (*E* points to the lateral and the middle cuneiform bones), middle (*5*) and medial (*4*) **cuneiform** bones are the other tarsal bones and articulate with the metatarsals (*F*) at the *tarsometatarsal joints*. The metatarsals articulate with the proximal phalanges (*G*) at the metatarsophalangeal joints. The great (big or first) toe has a proximal and distal phalanx; the remainder of the toes have proximal, middle, and distal phalanges.

The *lateral malleolus* is formed by the lateral distal aspect of the fibula and has a fossa on its posterior surface for the peroneus longus and brevis tendons. The *medial malleolus* is formed by the medial distal aspect of the tibia (tibia labeled *1*) and has a groove on its posterior surface for the tendons of the tibialis posterior and the flexor digitorum longus. Posterior to the medial malleolus, the pulse of the distal **posterior tibial artery,** which passes beneath the flexor retinaculum and lies between the flexor digitorum longus and the flexor hallicus longus, can be palpated.

The popliteal artery bifurcates just below the knee into the **anterior tibial artery** and the **tibioperoneal trunk,** which shortly thereafter bifurcates into the **posterior tibial** and **peroneal** arteries. The main terminal continuation of the anterior tibial artery is the **dorsalis pedis,** which begins anterior to the ankle, runs between the tendons of the extensor hallicus longus and extensor digitorum longus, and is palpable on the medial dorsal surface of the foot.

More High-Yield Facts

The *femoral artery* can be palpated at the level of the groin, midway between the anterior superior iliac spine and the symphysis pubis. From lateral to medial at the level the femoral artery is palpable run the femoral **n**erve, **a**rtery, **v**ein, an **e**mpty space (part of the femoral canal where femoral hernias occur), and **l**ymphatics (mnemonic: from lateral to medial, an arrow points toward the *NAVEL*). The *popliteal artery* can be palpated posterior to the knee in the popliteal fossa.

Case 46

Anatomy & Embryology

History

A 3-month-old infant is brought in by the mother for recurrent respiratory infections and chronic cough. The infant has had three respiratory infections since birth. Two of the prior episodes were pneumonia secondary to *Pseudomonas aeruginosa*. The mother also mentions that her infant is "salty tasting." The infant has had subnormal growth since birth. Family history includes a maternal aunt and paternal uncle who died at a young age from recurrent respiratory infections.

Physical Exam

The infant has a productive cough during the exam and rhonchi with bronchial breath sounds in the right lung. The infant coughs up tenacious, thick, green-tinged sputum. You notice visible salt crystals on the infant's skin, and she seems dehydrated.

Tests

Sweat analysis: increased levels of chloride
Serum trypsin: elevated
Chest x-ray: pneumonia in the right lung

Questions

- What condition is most likely responsible for the patient's symptoms?
- How is this condition inherited?
- What is the mechanism of disease in this condition?
- What organ systems are affected by this condition?

Topic Cystic fibrosis (CF)

Discussion

CF is an **autosomal recessive** disorder that results from a mutation in a gene on *chromosome 7* that codes for a **c-AMP-regulated transmembrane chloride transport protein** called **CFTR** (cystic fibrosis transmembrane conductance regulator). More than 600 different mutations have been identified, but 70% of cases are due to a deletion of three amino acids coding for phenylalanine (ΔF508 mutation).

The result is abnormally **thick secretions,** which affect the **sweat glands** and the **respiratory, gastrointestinal,** and **reproductive** systems. CF is the *most common lethal genetic disease in whites* (occurs in 1:3000 whites versus 1:15,000 in blacks). As a result of improved diagnosis and earlier and more effective treatment, patients with CF now **often live past 30.**

Findings

The classic history is a mother complaining of a **"salty tasting baby,"** which should immediately make you think of CF. Recurrent respiratory infections with *Staphylococcus aureus* and *Pseudomonas aeruginosa* are also classic. Chronic cough and failure to gain weight are common. Pancreatic insufficiency also frequently occurs and can lead to *diabetes mellitus* or **malabsorption** (especially of the fat-soluble vitamins A, D, E, and K) or both.

Diagnosis & Treatment

Diagnosis is made with the **sweat chloride test** (reveals elevated chloride concentration in sweat) and confirmed with **DNA probe** testing to identify the specific mutation, which has clinical and genetic counseling implications (CF can be detected in utero). Serum **trypsin** also is usually elevated in CF. Most cases are discovered during infancy. Treatment includes respiratory therapy, antibiotics, pancreatic enzyme replacement, and fat-soluble vitamin supplements.

More High-Yield Facts

Almost all men (vas deferens become obstructed with viscous material) and 50% of women with CF are *infertile*.

Patients eventually develop secondary **pulmonary hypertension** and right heart failure (**cor pulmonale**), and most eventually die of respiratory failure.

Other conditions that can develop in CF patients: **meconium ileus** (thick meconium causes bowel obstruction in the newborn) and **biliary cirrhosis** (bile ducts are chronically obstructed by thick mucinous material) with resultant portal hypertension and esophageal varices.

Case 47

Anatomy & Embryology

History

A 68-year-old man complains of arm weakness and dizziness when exercising. The man has known atherosclerotic disease and says his symptoms began a few months ago but have been getting worse. Whenever he uses his left arm for long periods his arm gets "tired" and painful, and he gets dizzy.

Physical Exam

The blood pressure in the left arm is 40 mmHg lower than in the right, and you hear a left supraclavicular bruit.

Tests

Angiogram: nearly complete occlusion at the origin of the left subclavian artery and reversed flow in the left vertebral artery

Subclavian and axillary arteries: see figure

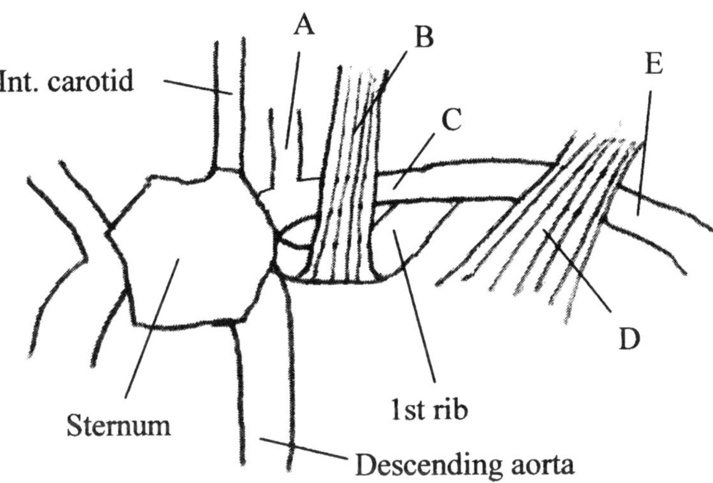

Questions

- Which labeled structure in the figure represents the vertebral artery?
- Which labeled structure in the figure is the axillary artery? The subclavian?
- Which labeled structures are the muscles that divide the subclavian and axillary arteries into their first, second, and third portions?
- What labeled artery supplies the first two posterior intercostal arteries?

Subclavian and axillary arteries

Discussion

The right subclavian artery arises from the *brachiocephalic trunk,* and the left arises directly from the *aortic arch*. The subclavian artery (labeled *C* in the figure) conventionally is divided into a first, second, and third portion by the **anterior scalene** muscle (*B*), which runs anterior to the subclavian. At the *lateral edge of the first rib,* which the subclavian runs over top of, the subclavian turns into the axillary artery.

The axillary artery (*E*) also is divided into three parts (first, second, and third) by the **pectoralis minor** muscle (*D*), which runs anterior to the artery to insert onto the coracoid process. The axillary artery ends at the *lower border of the teres minor muscle,* where it continues as the **brachial artery.** The branches of the axillary artery are as follows: highest thoracic artery (first portion), thoracoacromial and lateral thoracic artery (both from second portion), and subscapular and anterior and posterior humeral circumflex arteries from the third portion.

The major branches of the subclavian artery include the costocervical trunk, **vertebral artery** (*A*), internal thoracic artery, and thyrocervical trunk. The first two posterior intercostal arteries arise from the superior intercostal artery, which is a branch of the *costocervical trunk* from the subclavian. The subclavian and axillary veins travel *anteroinferior* to their respective arteries.

Findings

Because one of the first branches of the subclavian artery is the vertebral artery, occlusion of the proximal aspect of the subclavian artery (or the brachiocephalic trunk on the right) can result in reversal of flow within the vertebral artery as a means to supply blood to the arm. The clinical syndrome that results is known as **subclavian steal** and can result in arm weakness and pain (i.e., *claudication*) and symptoms of posterior circulation ischemia (e.g., dizziness, syncope) and *asymmetric blood pressures between the two upper extremities* or a supraclavicular bruit.

Treatment

Treatment of subclavian steal is usually surgery.

More High-Yield Facts

The brachial artery terminates by dividing into the **ulnar** and **radial** arteries, which course on the same side as their respective bones. The pulse of the brachial artery can be palpated *just above the medial aspect of the elbow* by pushing into the medial edge of the biceps muscle. The radial artery pulse can be felt on the radial side of the distal aspect of the wrist, and the ulnar artery can be palpated laterally at this same level.

Case 48

Anatomy & Embryology

History

A 22-year-old woman complains of constant runny and itchy nose and cough that gets worse every spring and summer. The patient's symptoms began years ago, but she has never sought medical attention for them. Her past medical history is otherwise unremarkable, and she takes no regular medications, although she says that over-the-counter antihistamines relieve her symptoms. Family history is positive for asthma.

Physical Exam

The patient has rhinitis and nasal and pharyngeal mucosal erythema, along with mild end-expiratory wheezing. You suspect allergies.

Tests

Cells seen on a peripheral blood smear: see figure

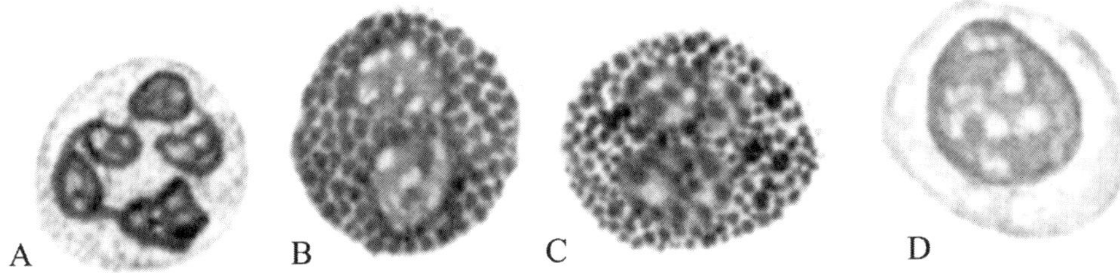

Questions

- Name the cell lettered *A,* the most abundant leukocyte in the blood.
- Name the cell lettered *B,* which has numerous reddish granules that contain major basic protein and is increased in number in this patient.
- Name the cell labeled *C,* which has numerous bluish granules that contain heparin and histamine.
- Name the cell labeled *D,* which can turn into a macrophage.

Topic Leukocytes

Discussion

Leukocytes, or white blood cells, are distinguished from red blood cells. There are six major categories of leukocytes found in the blood: neutrophils, eosinophils, basophils, monocytes, lymphocytes, and plasma cells (activated B lymphocytes). You should know the microscopic appearance of all of these cells before taking the USMLE step 1.

Findings

Neutrophils, eosinophils, and basophils all have nuclei with two or more lobes and are known as polymorphonuclear cells. All have distinct specific granules, and all are also known as granulocytes. **Neutrophils** (the cell labeled *A* in the figure) are the most numerous leukocyte found in the blood, comprising roughly 60% of the total. They are the first line of defense and the "workhorse" of the immune system, using phagocytosis to destroy bacteria and other foreign antigens.

Eosinophils (*B*) have granules that take up eosin and appear red on a hematoxylin and eosin–stained slide because the granules contain **major basic protein.** They are important in defending against parasitic infections (e.g., nematode infection). **Basophils** (*C* in the figure) have blue-staining granules that contain **histamine** and *heparin*. Basophils and **mast cells** are similar in function, but basophils circulate in the blood, while mast cells are fixed in tissue. Basophils can cause severe inflammation and systemic anaphylaxis when stimulated.

Monocytes (*D*) and lymphocytes (not shown) are agranulocytes, and their nuclei have only one lobe. Monocytes are the immature form of **macrophages** and circulate in the peripheral blood. When stimulated by inflammatory mediators, monocytes cross capillary walls and enter the connective tissues, where they differentiate into macrophages. Macrophages play a role in phagocytosis, antigen presentation, and cytokine production, especially *interleukin-1* and *tumor necrosis factor*. In the skin and subcutaneous tissues, fixed macrophages are known as **histiocytes,** whereas they are called **Kupffer cells** in the liver, **osteoclasts** in the bone, and **microglial cells** in the central nervous system.

More High-Yield Facts

Lymphocytes develop from a different stem cell (i.e., are of lymphocytic origin) than all other leukocytes, which are said to be of myelocytic origin. This is the reason leukemia is divided into the *lymphogenous* and *myelogenous* subtypes.

Case 49

Anatomy & Embryology

History

A 21-year-old woman comes to see you because she believes she is infertile. The woman has never menstruated and has been unable to conceive, although she has tried for the last 5 years. Her past medical and family history are unremarkable. The patient takes no medications and has never had any type of surgery.

Physical Exam

On pelvic exam, you are unable to palpate the uterus. The rest of the exam is unremarkable. MRI of the pelvis confirms that the uterus is absent.

Questions

- Match the adult structure with the embryonic structure from which it arises (the lettered answers can be used more than once or not at all):

1. Epididymis
2. Urinary bladder
3. Labia majora
4. Uterus
5. Seminal vesicles
6. Ureters

A. Labioscrotal folds
B. Paramesonephric ducts
C. Urogenital sinus
D. Mesonephric ducts
E. Gubernaculum

- Match the female structure with its embryologic male homologue (each lettered answer should be used once):

1. Skene's (paraurethral) glands
2. Labia majora
3. Glans penis
4. Bartholin's glands
5. Labia minora
6. Vagina and uterus
7. Gartner's duct
8. Testis

A. Prostatic utricle
B. Ovary
C. Ventral aspect of the penis
D. Cowper's (bulbourethral) glands
E. Clitoris
F. Prostate
G. Epididymis
H. Scrotum

Matching answers:
First question—1D, 2C, 3A, 4B, 5D, 6D
Second question—1F, 2H, 3E, 4D, 5C, 6A, 7G, 8B

Topic Genitourinary embryology

Discussion

The genitourinary system develops in tandem in a complex series of growth and regression of various structures, the pattern of which determines male versus female and errors in which can lead to various congenital anomalies.

In the male, the **mesonephric ducts** play a major role in reproductive organ formation, whereas in the female, the **paramesonephric ducts** are important (the less important ductal system almost completely regresses in both sexes).

Embryonic Structure	Male Derivative(s)	Female Derivative(s)
Mesonephric tubules and ducts*	Epididymis, vas deferens, seminal vesicles, ejaculatory duct	Gartner's duct, epoöphoron, paroöphoron
Paramesonephric ducts	Appendix of testicle, prostatic utricle	Uterus, cervix, fallopian tubes, upper one third of vagina
Urogenital sinus†	Prostate gland, Cowper's glands	Vagina, urethra, Skene's glands, Bartholin's glands
Genital tubercle/phallus	Penis	Clitoris
Urogenital/urethral folds	Ventral aspect of the penis	Labia minora
Labioscrotal folds (i.e., genital swellings)	Scrotum	Labia majora

*The mesonephric ducts also indirectly form the ureters and renal collecting systems in both sexes via the ureteric bud, an outgrowth of the mesonephric duct.
†The urogenital sinus also gives rise to the urinary bladder and urethra in both sexes.

Male and Female Homologues

Male Structure	Female Structure
Testes	Ovaries
Epididymis	Gartner's duct
Prostatic utricle	Uterus and vagina
Prostate gland	Skene's (paraurethral) glands
Cowper's (bulbourethral) glands	Bartholin's (greater vestibular) glands
Penis	Clitoris
Ventral aspect of the penis	Labia minora
Scrotum	Labia majora

More High-Yield Facts

The Y chromosome contains a gene that codes for **testes-determining factor,** which cause the gonads to turn into testes. When testes-determining factor is absent, ovaries are formed. Sertoli cells of the testes secrete **müllerian-inhibiting factor,** which causes the paramesonephric ducts to regress. In the absence of müllerian-inhibiting factor, the paramesonephric ducts persist and form female structures.

Further work-up would be required to determine the specific abnormality in this patient. One possibility is testicular feminization syndrome (i.e., androgen insensitivity), which results in an XY karyotype with a female phenotype (e.g., breast tissue, enlarged clitoris, vagina). Those affected lack a uterus and ovaries and thus never menstruate (the syndrome is a cause of primary amenorrhea).

Case 50

Anatomy & Embryology

History

A 2-year-old child is brought to the emergency department with abdominal pain and vomiting that began yesterday and have been getting worse. The patient has no significant past medical history, was previously healthy, and takes no medications. Family history is unremarkable.

Physical Exam

The patient has abdominal tenderness, and an x-ray of the abdomen is suspicious for bowel obstruction. The patient is taken to the operating room, and the surgeon makes a midline incision to gain exposure to the peritoneal cavity. The surgeon finds that there is bowel obstruction, which seems to be related to an abnormal outpouching from the distal ileum that is connected to the anterior abdominal wall by a fibrous cord (see figure).

Tests

Electrolytes: normal

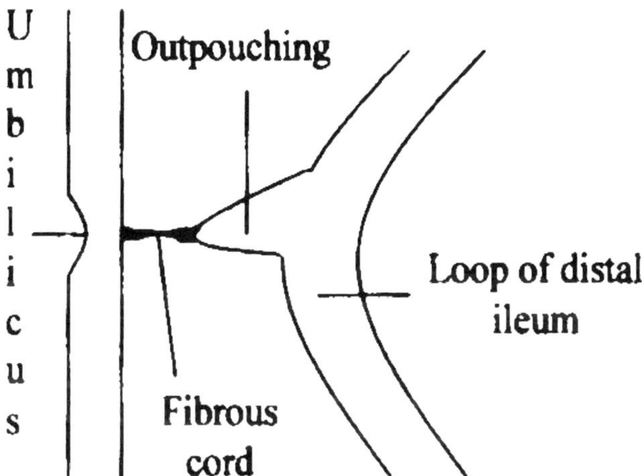

Questions

- What is the clinical name of this outpouching?
- What embryologic structure does it arise from? What two things does this structure connect in utero?
- How common is it, and where does it typically occur?
- What problems can this embryologic remnant cause?

Meckel's diverticulum (MD)

Discussion

MD is a remnant of the **vitelline duct.** In utero, this structure connects the *midgut* and the **yolk sac** and, along with the *connecting stalk* (which eventually develops into the true umbilical cord), passes through the *umbilical ring* and helps to form the **primitive umbilical cord.** Normally the yolk sac regresses or obliterates in utero.

In roughly **2%** of the population, MD occurs, which typically is found within **2** feet of the ileocecal valve on the *antimesenteric side of the distal ileum.* Many patients are asymptomatic, but symptoms often come to medical attention by age **2** years; symptoms are twice as common in males. All of these "2s" add up to the *rule of twos* for MD.

Findings

Patients can have *bowel obstruction,* especially when there is a fibrous band that connects the MD to the abdominal wall, as in this patient. MD also can contain heterotopic (i.e., normal tissue in the wrong place) *gastric mucosa,* in which case it can lead to bleeding, ulceration, and perforation.

With complete persistence of the vitelline duct, a *vitelline or umbilical fistula* is said to be present, which can lead to **fecal discharge at the umbilicus.**

Treatment

Treatment for such a fistula or a symptomatic MD is surgery. Most cases of MD are asymptomatic and require no treatment.

More High-Yield Facts

Physiologic herniation of the midgut outside the abdominal cavity occurs in utero during the first trimester. The loops come back into the abdominal cavity and rotate **270° counterclockwise** to form the normal bowel relationships in the adult. **Malrotation** can occur if the loops fail to rotate or do not rotate enough, leading to an abnormal relationship of the segments of the bowel (e.g., cecum on the left instead of the right).

An **omphalocele** occurs when intestinal loops fail to return to the abdominal cavity in utero. At birth, the herniated loops can be seen at the abdominal wall surface as a large swelling within the umbilical cord. The loops are covered only by amnion (no skin or abdominal wall muscles cover the loops). Treatment is surgery to put the loops back within the peritoneal cavity.

FIGURE CREDITS

Case 1
Both figures from Mettler FA Jr: Head and soft tissues of the neck. In Essentials of Radiology. Philadelphia, W.B. Saunders, 1996; with permission.

Case 2
From Wood ME (ed): Hematology/Oncology Secrets, 2nd ed (color panels). Philadelphia, Hanley & Belfus, 1999; with permission.

Case 4
Modified from Schoen FJ: The heart. In Cotran RS et al (eds): Robbins Pathologic Basis of Disease, 5th ed. Philadelphia, W.B. Saunders, 1994.

Case 5
From Brochert A: Crush Step 3. Philadelphia, Hanley & Belfus, 2001, p 79; with permission.

Case 7
From Mettler FA Jr: The skeletal system. In Essentials of Radiology. Philadelphia, W.B. Saunders, 1996; with permission.

Case 9
From Concannon MJ: Hand anatomy. In Common Hand Problems in Primary Care. Philadelphia, Hanley & Belfus, Inc., 1999, p 10; with permission.

Case 12
From Kumar V: Genetic disorders. In Cotran RS et al (eds): Robbins Pathologic Basis of Disease, 5th ed. Philadelphia, W.B. Saunders, 1994; with permission.

Case 13
From Torma MJ, Wade TP, James ED: Liver, biliary tract, and pancreas. In James EC, Corry RJ, Perry JF (eds): Principles of Basic Surgical Practice. Philadelphia, Hanley & Belfus, 1987; with permission.

Case 15
From Heydorn WH: Abdominal hernia. In James EC, Corry RJ, Perry JF (eds): Principles of Basic Surgical Practice. Philadelphia, Hanley & Belfus, 1987; with permission.

Case 17
From Silver RM, Smith EA: Rheumatology Pearls. Philadelphia, Hanley & Belfus, 1997, p 71; with permission.

Case 18

From Disorders of nerve and muscle. In Forbes CD, Jackson WF (eds): Color Atlas and Text of Clinical Medicine. London, Mosby-Wolfe, 1993; with permission.

Case 21

From Wilhite JM: Thoracic and lumbosacral spine. In Mellion MB, et al (eds): Team Physician's Handbook, 3rd ed. Philadelphia, Hanley & Belfus, 2002, p 460; with permission.

Case 23

From Guyton AC: Heart sounds: Dynamics of valvular and congenital heart defects. In Guyton Textbook of Physiology, 8th ed. Philadelphia, WB Saunders, 1991, p 259; with permission.

Case 25

From Nienhuis AW, Wolfe L: The thalassemias. In Nathan DG, Oski FA (eds): Hematology of Infancy and Childhood, 3rd ed. Philadelphia, WB Saunders, 1987, p 735; with permission.

Case 32

From Fitzpatrick JE, Aeling JL (eds): Dermatology Secrets (color panels). Philadelphia, Hanley & Belfus, 1996; with permission.

Case 41

From Martinez-Frontanilla LA: Tracheoesophageal malformations. In Harken AH, Moore EE (eds): Abernathy's Surgical Secrets, 3rd ed. Philadelphia, Hanley & Belfus, 1996, p 271–274; with permission.

Case 42

From Tu HK, Davis LF, Nique TA: Maxillofacial injuries. In Mellion MB, et al (eds): Team Physician's Handbook, 3rd ed. Philadelphia, Hanley & Belfus, 2002, p 392; with permission.

Case 45

From Hunter SC, DeLoach JG, McLean RB: Foot problems. In Mellion MB, et al (eds): Team Physician's Handbook, 3rd ed. Philadelphia, Hanley & Belfus, 2002, p 536; with permission.

Case 48

From Guyton AC: Blood cells, immunity, and blood clotting. In Guyton Textbook of Physiology, 8th ed. Philadelphia, WB Saunders, 1991, p 366; with permission.

CASE INDEX

Notes

Notes

Notes

Notes

Notes

Notes

Notes

Notes

Notes

Notes

Notes

Notes